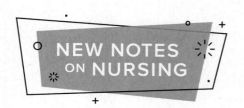

SUCCESSFUL STUDYING
FOR NURSING STUDENTS

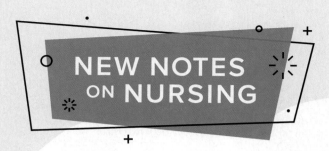

NEW NOTES ON NURSING

SUCCESSFUL STUDYING FOR NURSING STUDENTS

EDITOR

Melanie Hayward, RN
Child, RSN SCPHN, CPNP,
RNT, DipHe, Grad Cert,
BSc (Hons), PGDip, MAEd,
FHEA, FRSA

SERIES EDITOR

Teresa Chinn, MBE,
RN, QN

CONSULTING EDITOR

June Girvin

ELSEVIER

Notices

Practitioners and researchers must always rely on their own experience and knowledge in evaluating and using any information, methods, compounds or experiments described herein. Because of rapid advances in the medical sciences, in particular, independent verification of diagnoses and drug dosages should be made. To the fullest extent of the law, no responsibility is assumed by Elsevier, authors, editors or contributors for any injury and/or damage to persons or property as a matter of products liability, negligence or otherwise, or from any use or operation of any methods, products, instructions, or ideas contained in the material herein.

ISBN: 978-0-443-10711-5

Printed in India

Last digit is the print number: 9 8 7 6 5 4 3 2 1

Content Strategist: Robert Edwards
Content Project Manager: Shivani Pal
Design: Renee Duenow

Working together
to grow libraries in
developing countries

www.elsevier.com • www.bookaid.org

CONTRIBUTORS

Rebecca Boden, RN (Child), Dip HE, BSc (Hons), PGCHPE, FHEA.

Jennie Brady, RN (Child), BSc (Hons), BA (Hons).

Victoria Carter, RN Adult, RHV SCPHN, MSc.

Andrea Cockett RN Child/Adult, RNT, BSc (Hons), EdD, MA, PGDHE, SFHEA

Fi Croucher RGN, RSCN, MSc, BSc, FHEA

Fiona Cust, RN (Adult), RN (Child), RHV SCPHN, PGDipHPE, DHSci, SFHEA.

Catherine Forward, RN Adult, RSN SCPHN, BA, MML, SFHEA

Charlotte Jakab-Hall, RN Adult, FHEA, PGCAP, BSc (Hons), BA (Hons)

Anita Z Goldschmied, RN (Learning Disabilities), BA (Hons), PgCert Ed., PgDip Mgmt, MRes, PhD FHEA

Jennifer Hanley, RN Child, PgCert, BSc (Hons)

Phill Hoddinott, RN (Adult), DipHE, BSc, PGCE/RNT, MSc, DIC, SFHEA

Dean-David Holyoake, RN (Mental Health), Dip CPC, Dip Child Psychol, BSc (Hons), BA, PgCert Ed, PG Dip N, MSc, PhD, SFHEA

Sophie Kempshall, RN (Child), PGCHPE, FHEA

Rachael Major, RN Adult, RNT, DipHE, BSc(Hons), MA, EdD, SFHEA, FSET, MILoL

Cathryn Peppard, MA, FHEA

Debbie Roberts, RN Adult. PhD, PFHEA.

Julia Williams, RN, Dip D/N, BSc (Hons), MA Ed, PhD, SFHEA

CONTENTS

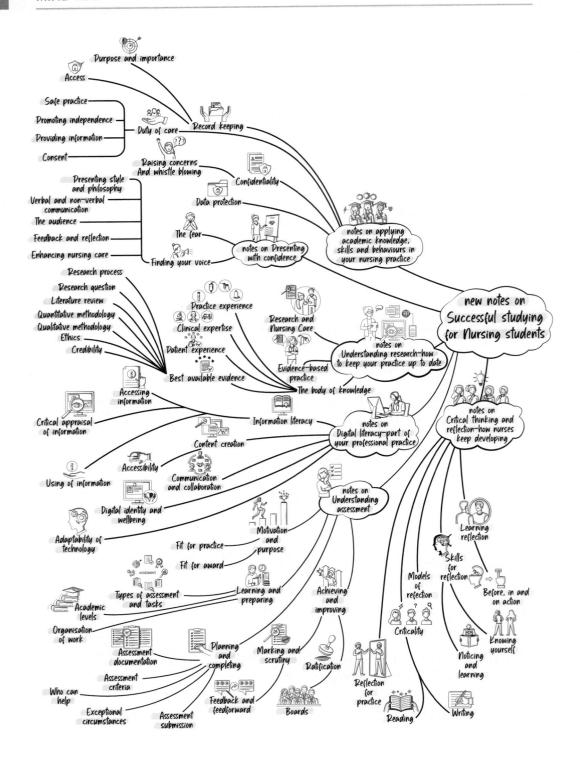

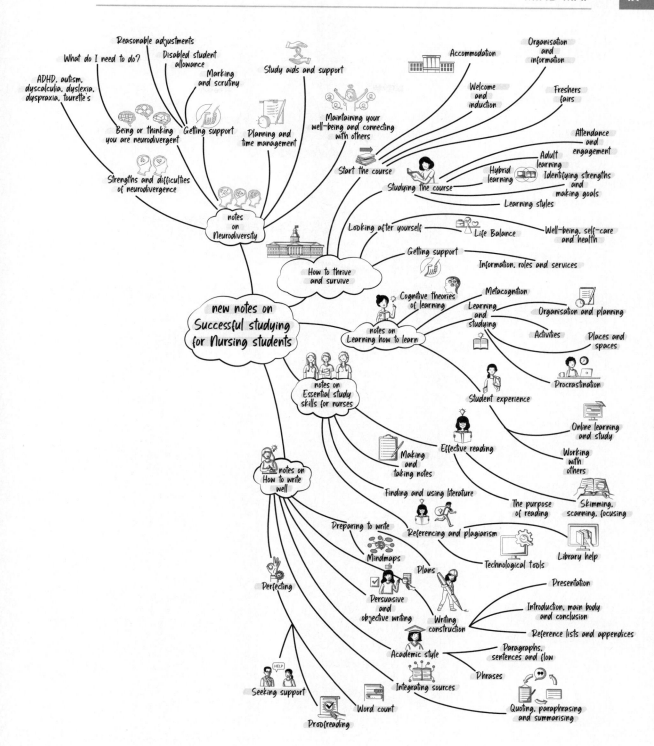

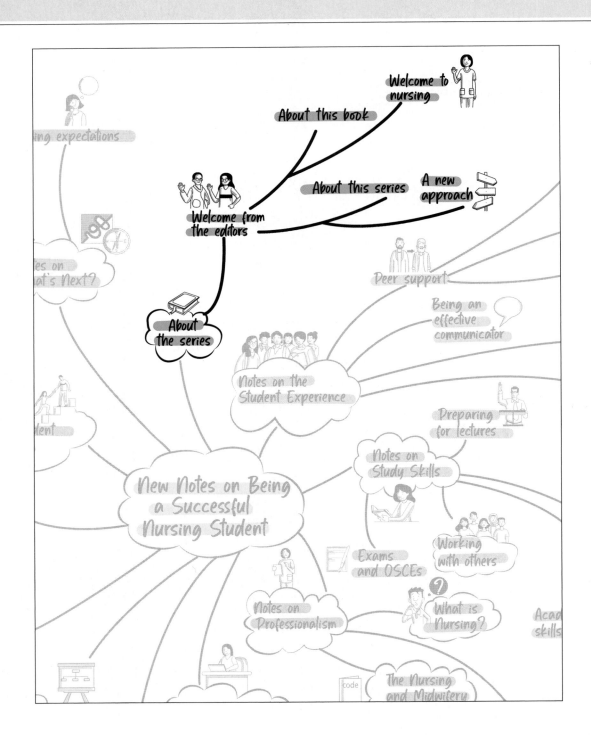

ABOUT THIS SERIES

Teresa Chinn (She/Her) ■ **June Girvin (She/Her)**

DEAR NURSING STUDENT,

We are so pleased that you have chose this book from the other nursing books on the shelf! You may have noticed that it looks a little different to other books in the nursing section and there's a very good reason for that – it is different! This is the first in a series of books aimed at supporting you as a nursing student. The series combines a nursing book and a digital perspective, including the use of social media, that we hope will create a user-friendly and engaging approach to some of the fundamental topics and challenges in nursing.

The title for the series *New Notes on Nursing* is respectfully and humbly borrowed from Florence Nightingale's own writing. Her *Notes on Nursing* (1860), outlined a vision for health and wellness that encompassed social, political, economic and environmental determinants as well as public health and illness prevention – the bigger picture within which good nursing care must be grounded. We recognise that for many new nursing students, some of the concepts that inform nursing can be challenging and complex, and may not always appear immediately relevant. The *New Notes...* series seeks to address that. We have tried hard to present content in a friendly style, conversational as far as possible, and incorporating social media so that interacting with this book is not a solitary activity but one that can be shared with others who are using the same book and finding out about the same things – whether they are in your cohort or somewhere else in the United Kingdom.

We are trying new design approaches using colourful and engaging content that is aimed at helping you identify the information you need quickly and easily. We understand that sometimes you don't want (or need) to read a dense textbook from start to finish to pull out the most helpful information for your situation, but rather easily identify the bits that are relevant for you at a point in time. We think our colour-coding and infographics throughout the books will help you do just that. We have also included all sorts of helpful 'sidenotes'; again taking inspiration from Florence Nightingale's writing:

THE NMC SAYS

These show the part of the code that the text is relevant to, helping you to embed the code into every area of your practice and thinking.

SOCIAL MEDIA

'These are tweets from Registered Nurses and nursing students that share snippets of wisdom and perspective'

We have asked many people to contribute to the New Notes on Nursing books and we have included some long quotes from these people; these have been especially written for this series.

CASE STUDY

Case studies, both real and imagined, are a great way to put learning into context, so you will find plenty of them in this series.

Your notes are just as important as ours and you will find lots of space in *New Notes on Nursing* for your own notes.

_____

_____

_____

_____

_____

_____

_____

_____

We have created the books with neurodiversity in mind and have tried to ensure that there is a feeling of space and lightness to the book.

In addition to all of this, we really want to engage and support you on your nursing student journey, so we have created some social media resources for you to tap into. Please search #NewNotesOnNursing and #SuccessfulStN on SOCIAL MEDIA to find out more.

The team of Editors and Authors that we have asked to contribute to *New Notes on Nursing* are all practising health and care professionals, ranging in experience from nursing students and newly qualified Registered Nurses to registered professionals working in clinical and education settings with a wealth of experience. They all wanted to help you. By inviting a variety of voices to create these books, we are sharing many perspectives with you. We hope it helps you to develop well-rounded views on which to start your nursing career.

You are the latest generation of nursing students, and we are so pleased and honoured to be, in some small way, supporting you to flourish. We really hope you enjoy this book (yes, enjoy!) and that, at the end of your student journey, it contains lots of notes scribbled by you, the pages are dog-eared and the cover well-worn – a new generation of nursing texts for a new generation of Registered Nurses.

Today's nursing is socially complex, politically enmeshed and at times finding its way through conflict and controversy to give the best holistic, person-centred care. We think it's the best career in the world.

Best wishes

June and Teresa

The series is edited by:

'I've been a Registered Nurse since 1996 and have made my career in the social care sector. In 2012 set up the nursing Twitter community @WeNurses to help bring together nurses from diverse spheres of practice. I was awarded an MBE for services to nursing in 2014 and in 2018, I was named one of the 70 most influential nurses from 1948 to 2018 by the Royal College of Nursing. I communicate in many different ways in the UK and Europe, particularly on the use of social media in Nursing. I was made a Queens Nurse in 2022'.

Teresa Chinn, MBE QN @WeNurses

'I qualified as a Registered Nurse in 1976 and have spent a (very) long career in clinical and academic practice. I retired in 2017 and now work independently in roles committed to supporting individual nurses and nursing as a profession – writing, commentating, coaching, reviewing, etc. I was delighted to be asked to support the development of this new series of books and to work with the team of writers/editors and Elsevier'.

June Girvin @ProfJuneG

REFERENCES

Nightingale, Florence. 1860. Notes on nursing: what it is, and what it is not. London: Harrison. Harvard (18th ed.).

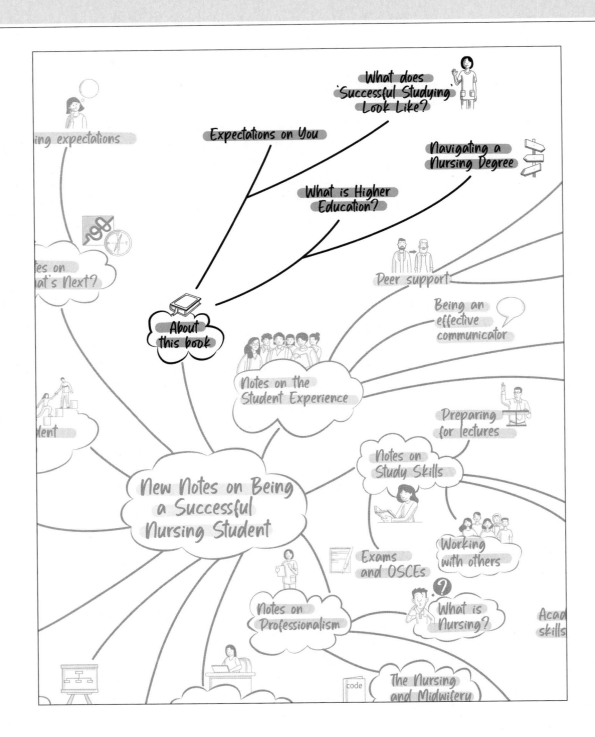

ABOUT THIS BOOK

Melanie Hayward (She/Her)

HEY THERE, FUTURE NURSES!

Welcome to "Successful Studying for Nursing Students," the second book in our New Notes on Nursing series. Studying to be a nurse isn't a walk in the park; it's a rollercoaster of emotions filled with challenge and celebration!

Now, what makes our book stand out from other books about studying nursing? Well, buckle up — it's not your typical nursing read. We've teamed up with some amazing authors, and what's cooler is nursing students and newly registered nurses who've been in your shoes not too long ago have contributed to many chapters. So, the information you're getting is not just textbook stuff; it's real, relatable, and laser-focused on what you need to ace your pre-registration nursing studies. It's not just a book; it's your trusty sidekick!

So, what is it all about?

"Successful Studying for Nursing Students," unfolds as a crucial roadmap for your academic journey. Begin with insights into university life, discovering not just how to survive but to thrive in the challenging environment. Delve into the art of efficient learning, mastering study skills tailored to the unique demands of nursing education. The journey continues with chapters dedicated to crafting articulate written communication, cultivating critical thinking, and navigating diverse assessment methods. Explore the realm of digital literacy crucial for contemporary nursing practice, and gain insights into staying at the forefront of evidence-based care through understanding research. Develop confident presentation skills, essential for advocacy and leadership in nursing. Seamlessly integrate academic knowledge into practical nursing applications, bridging the gap between theory and real-world practice. The exploration concludes with a deep dive into neurodiversity, fostering an inclusive and understanding environment within the diverse landscape of nursing education.

But, first, let's begin by demystifying what higher education means for you and what expectations lie ahead.

What is Higher Education?

In a nutshell, higher education is the next level of academic exploration beyond secondary school. It's a space where you'll deepen your understanding of nursing, broaden your critical thinking skills, and cultivate the expertise needed to become a Registered Nurse. This isn't just about textbooks and exams; it's an immersive experience where you'll engage with fellow students, collaborate with experienced educators, work and learn from registered nurses and other qualified professionals in practice or the workplace, and actively participate in your learning journey.

Expectations on You

Now, let's consider what's expected from you in this exciting academic venture. Your pre-registration nursing degree programme demands dedication, curiosity, and a willingness to embrace challenges. It's not just about memorising facts; it's about applying theoretical knowledge to real-world scenarios. Active participation in classes, reflectiveness and open-mindedness to diverse perspectives, and a commitment to your personal and professional growth are key.

Navigating a Pre-Registration Nursing Degree Programme:

Successfully navigating a pre-registration nursing degree programme involves:

1. **Engagement:** Actively participating in lectures, seminars, and skills and simulation sessions. Your engagement fosters a deeper understanding of nursing concepts.
2. **Critical thinking:** Embrace the art of critical thinking. Question, analyse, and evaluate information. This skill is your compass in the world of nursing.
3. **Practice learning:** Your academic journey extends beyond the classroom. Embrace a variety of placements and work-based learning, it is imperative to apply theory to real patient care.
4. **Self-Care:** Balancing academic demands with self-care is crucial. Know when to take a break, seek support when needed, and prioritise your well-being.

So, what does 'Successful Studying' Look Like?

Success in your studies goes beyond grades. It's about:

1. **Understanding:** Grasping nursing concepts and understanding their practical applications.
2. **Resilience:** Navigating challenges with resilience, bouncing back from setbacks, and using them as learning opportunities.
3. **Reflective practice:** Continuously reflecting on your experiences, identifying areas for improvement or celebration, and evolving as a nursing student.
4. **Community:** Building a supportive community with your peers, educators and healthcare professionals. This may be at your university, where you live, in practice or even virtually through online groups and social media. Collaboration enhances your learning journey.

TIPS

- Participate actively in lectures, seminars, skills and simulation sessions. Engage with the learning material to deepen your understanding.
- Create a study routine that suits your learning style. Break down complex topics, set realistic goals, and review regularly.
- Ask questions. Whether it's in class, during placements, or in study groups or tutorials, seeking clarification enhances your comprehension.
- Connect with fellow nursing students. Form study groups, share experiences, and support each other through the ups and downs of the programme.
- Regularly reflect on your experiences – both in theory and practice learning. Identify areas for improvement and celebrate successes.
- Ensure you get enough rest, maintain a healthy lifestyle, and seek support when needed.
- Take advantage of the resources available to you – library materials, online databases, and academic support services. They are there to enhance your learning.
- Keep track of assessments, deadlines, and shift patterns. Staying organised will help reduce stress and ensure you meet all your commitments.
- Attend online webinars, networking events, conferences and career fairs. Building connections with experienced professionals can provide insights and open doors to future opportunities.
- Acknowledge and celebrate your achievements, whether big or small. Completing assignments, mastering a new skill, or successfully completing a placement – every step counts!

Before you start delving into each chapter – have a go at this reflective exercise and start to chart your 'Studying for Nursing' journey.

- Write down your **motivations** for pursuing nursing, the challenges you anticipate, and what success in your studies looks like to you.
- Reflect on your **expectations**. List three personal commitments you are willing to make to meet these expectations, considering dedication, curiosity and embracing challenges.
- Create a visual representation (chart, mind map or timeline) of your **envisioned journey** through the pre-registration nursing degree programme. Highlight key milestones, potential challenges, and areas where you anticipate personal and professional growth.
- In response to the four elements of **success** – Understanding, Resilience, Reflective Practice, and Community – jot down specific actions or strategies you plan to implement to embody each of these aspects in your academic journey.
- Choose three **tips** from the provided list that resonate most with you. Write a short paragraph explaining how you plan to incorporate these tips into your study routine or daily life as a nursing student.
- Conclude your reflective activity with a brief paragraph summarising your **key takeaways** from this introduction. Consider how this reflective exercise has shaped your mindset as you embark on learning how to be successful in your nursing studies.

_____

_____

_____

_____

Remember, this activity is a personal exploration, and there are no right or wrong answers. It's a tool for self-discovery, goal setting, and envisioning your unique 'Studying for Nursing' journey.

And finally......

Your nursing education extends far beyond the completion of your course; it marks the beginning of a perpetual learning journey. In the ever-evolving landscape of nursing and healthcare, where advancements and discoveries continually shape our practice, a commitment to continuous learning becomes imperative. Transitioning from nursing student to a registered nurse, the study skills and habits honed during your pre-registration nursing degree programme become invaluable, evolving into lifelong tools for staying current with evidence-based practices, embracing new technologies, and adapting to the dynamic healthcare environment. Your journey as a compassionate and competent nurse unfolds as an ongoing narrative, where every patient encounter and each challenge become an opportunity for learning and growth. Remember, these study skills are not confined to this course but are your allies throughout your entire career.

Best of luck as you embark on this journey of knowledge and growth. Do connect with me on X, my handle is @melhayward and share your journey using the hashtag **#SuccessfulStudying**. Your successes, big or small, are worth celebrating, and I look forward to reading all about them.

Warm wishes

Mel

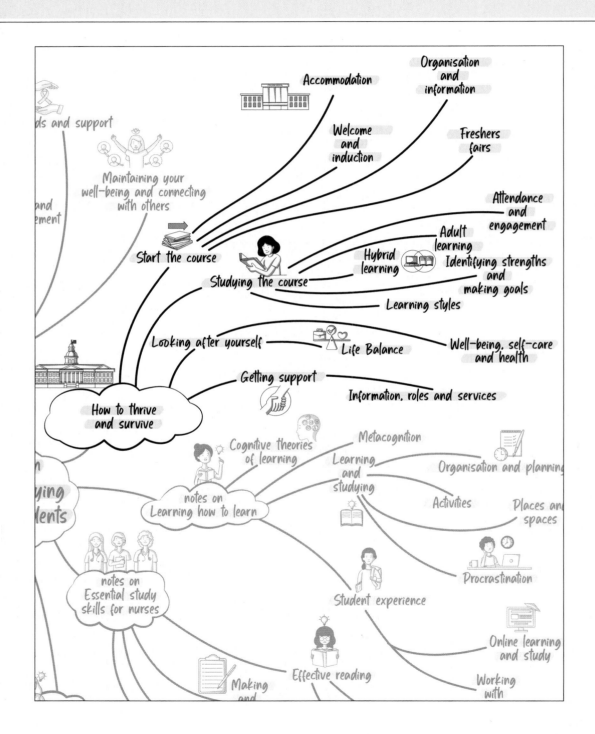

HOW TO THRIVE AND SURVIVE

Jennifer Hanley (she/her) ∎ **Phill Hoddinott (he/him)**

INTRODUCTION

Going to university is an exciting prospect, particularly when starting on a professional course. However, adjusting to university life within adult higher education may feel daunting and challenging, particularly during the first year of study on a nursing course.

This chapter aims to explore many areas to help you prepare for your first year of your nursing course at university. This will include what you need to do to thrive and survive at university. It will help you to explore your adult learning style as well as identify the support and well-being services that can help you, particularly during challenging times.

These areas will be further explored using case studies to help you reflect on your own experiences as well as prepare you for challenges that you might encounter, and you will be invited to make notes around your own reflections at the end of this chapter.

STARTING A NURSING COURSE AT UNIVERSITY

Congratulations on starting your nursing course at university. Whether you are new to adult higher education or you have previously studied at university, you will have put in a lot of hard work to get here; welcome to the beginning of your nursing journey.

Starting university is an exciting, life-changing event but can sometimes feel daunting. Nursing students often report feelings attached to imposter syndrome. This includes feelings of inadequacy, self-doubt and anxiety that can have a catastrophic effect on the personal and professional development of your student journey (Atkinson, 2022).

Knowing what to expect, planning your time and completing everything you need to in a timely manner will help you to get your nursing journey off to the best start. Making new friends and building support networks will make this journey even better and will help you with your transition into studying nursing at university.

Accommodation

For some, starting university might mean you are leaving home for the first time or relocating to another area. For others, you may have chosen to study closer to home. You may have prearranged to move into university accommodation, often referred to as 'halls', or you may be renting privately to start at university. It is important that you plan this carefully and take time to find the right place to live.

Living in university accommodation is usually the cheaper option and can be fun, but you might find yourself sharing living accommodation with other students. This often means that you will share common living spaces such as kitchens, bathrooms and lounges, but you will usually have your own room where you can sleep and study. Remember that your home is a place for you to relax as well as study independently, so finding some quiet time can often be a challenge for new students. Learning who manages the accommodation is important so you can get help and support should you need it, and perhaps when getting to know your neighbours, you can start to agree on some ground rules or 'ways of living together'. Remember, as a nursing student, you will be engaging in practice learning, and this will mean doing shift work that could involve being on clinical placements during unsocial hours (nights, weekends and bank holidays), so being able to rest and sleep is important.

Many universities will have an accommodation department that can help students to find accommodation and support students with accommodation concerns, find out where they are based and what services they offer.

Living on your own or in shared accommodation is often preferred by many people, as it can feel more homely, and you may live with fewer people or your own family. Renting privately can be costly compared to university accommodation, and you must make sure that you have access to funds in order to be able to pay your rent and bills.

 TIP

Students on a nursing course will have access to the NHS Learning Support Fund. You can find out more information about it via their website at www.nhsbsa.nhs.uk/nhs-learning-support-fund-lsf.

Find out from the university accommodation department about the support they can give to their students around private renting. Make sure that you are aware of all reductions and discounts on utility and other bills that you might be entitled to.

 TIP

Many businesses offer student discounts and have offers on utilities like broadband and mobile phone contracts, so do not forget to ask the students' union about this.

Welcoming you to university

Your university will have worked hard to welcome all their new students. Whilst most students start university in September, sometimes nursing courses begin outside of the usual academic year, so some activities may differ.

University and course induction

In the first week of your university course, you will be given lots of information; this can often feel overwhelming, but it is an important introduction and will cover a lot of administrative processes that need to be completed. Topics around how the course is delivered, placement information, university attendance and expectations will be covered. Information around pastoral support, as well as university wellness and other support mechanisms, will also be introduced.

Getting organised

Planning and organisation will be an important part of your success in your nursing course. Getting into good habits from the start of your course will be beneficial to you.

There will be several administrative tasks that you need to do in order to successfully enrol on your course; these could include:

- University enrolment processes, including proof of previous study and the right to study in the United Kingdom
- Student finance registration

As a nursing student, you will have to do some further administrative processes that many other students may not usually be required to do.

NMC

THE NMC SAYS

1 Guidance on health and character says
'Better and safer care for people is at the heart of what we do. We make sure that only those who meet our requirements are allowed to practise as a nurse or midwife in the UK, or a nursing associate in England.'

This is a requirement of the Nursing and Midwifery Council (NMC), which is detailed further in their guidance of health and character (NMC, 2019). This could include:

- Signing a 'Directional Statement' or student agreement around adhering to not only the university regulations, but it also covers professional issues around being a student in an NMC-regulated course
- Choosing or giving a preference for a clinical placement area

- Ordering and collecting your uniform, badge and student identification
- Obtaining occupational health or health clearance
- Having a police check known as Disclosure and Barring Service

These processes are important, and not completing them in a timely manner may delay or even jeopardise your progression in the course. You must understand what you need to do, when you need to submit it by, where you need to submit it, when you need to do and, most importantly, what it says.

Course information

One of the most important things you can do to reduce anxiety or uncertainty is to access and read the key documents and sections of your virtual learning environment (e.g., BlackBoard, Moodle) which outline the upcoming course expectations.

NMC

THE NMC SAYS

3.2 'Students are provided with timely and accurate information about curriculum, approaches to teaching, supervision, assessment, practice placements and other information relevant to their course'.

This information should be available to you at the start of the course and/or modules or units of learning you are currently undertaking. The documents outlining this information should be student-friendly and accessible. These will likely include:

- **Programme or course handbook** is an essential read. This will tell you everything you need not know about the course and will have lots of information around health and safety, expectations and professional values, as well as support mechanisms.
- **Practice or placement handbook** contains an overview of placement expectations, student responsibilities, practice learning, supervision and assessment processes.

- **Course schedule or plan** sets out what each year or part of your course looks like. This is particularly relevant to you as a nursing student, as your course may look different from other courses. Details of when you are expected to be at university, when you are on placement and when your holidays are will all be helpful.
- **Timetable** will break down your weekly teaching and learning activities and will give you details of days/timings of taught sessions, where these are held (remember that many universities now offer a hybrid teaching and learning, so you may have a mixture of online and face-to-face teaching) and who will be running these.

You will be given information about the modules/units that you will be studying. This will include the time requirements for teaching and learning, indicative content, reading list and the learning outcomes. Details of the assessment(s) will also be outlined. You may also be given further information about the assessment within a separate briefing document.

TIP

In the reflection space at the end of this chapter space, record the documents you were given access to during your first week on the course, or consider any questions you may have for the lecturers about these documents.

Freshers' fairs

Becoming a learner on a healthcare professional-regulated course and being a nursing student are unique experiences. The design of your course and the way you study and learn may be very different compared to other courses that your university offers. It is, however, important to recognise yourself as a student and to explore university life outside of the nursing school, department or division.

Freshers' fairs are a good opportunity to discover what the wider university offers. You will be able to find out more information about central university services such as well-being support, accommodation office and central student life services. The students' union (SU) is often a useful source of support, from representation and personal support to social activities and offers to join societies. Many student societies are already established, but the SU often will help students to set up their own society.

CASE STUDY

Pramila is a mature student and has not studied for many years. She lives at home with her husband and two teenage sons. Pramila feels excited to be pursuing a nursing career and to be back at university after so many years of working and being at home with her family. After attending the first-day induction, Pramila feels anxious about the amount of information that has been given, particularly around the hybrid learning timetable and the submission dates. Pramila's main worry is that she will miss the submission dates and fail the whole course.

What would you suggest to Pramila?

[Our suggestion] It is usual to feel overwhelmed by starting something new. Being organised needs to be every student's new best friend. Remember, there will always be people on the course, at the university and in the student centre that are there to help, support and signpost you, so always ask for help.

Reading the course handbook and all the other documentation already discussed in this section will often answer many questions students have. Taking time to sit down and read these is important. Reading in bite-size chunks, little and often, and making notes can often be helpful. Some people find reading and retaining information difficult, so using technology that will read this aloud could be helpful.

TIP

Buy a paper diary or use an electronic diary so you can input all the key dates to help you organise your life balance around your nursing course. Using a wall planner or calendar could help you focus on the important dates and will act as a more visual aid.

SOCIAL MEDIA
@AmyPile4

'Remember, we are all different and have different commitments, have a diary, set aside time, be realistic, you need to be honest with yourself and know your limitations, but you won't know until you try, it's definitely something you learn along the way'

CASE STUDY

Ben finished his A levels over the summer and has started his nursing course at university in September. Ben comes from a small village and has left home for the first time. Ben is living in university student halls and has a room on a floor that houses 11 other students. Ben is very quiet and shy and is finding it difficult to come out of his room to socialise with people he does not know, as he does not know what to say. He sat next to someone during the first day of the induction and got on quite well with them, but he lives in another student hall building. Ben is worried that he will not make any friends.

What would you suggest to Ben?

[Our suggestion] Moving away from home and starting university is exciting, but for some, it can be challenging, and adjusting to university life is not always straightforward. Finding a friendship and peer support network is important. Some people find this on their course, through their accommodation or through other channels within the university.

It is great that Ben has found someone he can talk to on the course, and perhaps he could suggest meeting up with this person outside of the course timetable. Networking is often a very good way to meet people, and friends of friends can often be a good way to further expand your friendship circle. Is there a social media platform for your course or cohort? This is often a good way to start networking with people on your course and arrange social events, for example.

Going to the freshers' fair could also help Ben to find activities to meet friends. Many SU organisations have organised societies and

CASE STUDY—cont'd

hold activities. Most universities have an SU presence on most campuses that can offer help and advice as well as signposting. Ben can call in and find out what they have to offer and perhaps even consider joining the SU as a volunteer.

STUDYING A NURSING COURSE AT UNIVERSITY

When starting a nursing course at university, it is important to be aware of how the course is likely to run and what you can do to help you prepare yourself for the journey ahead. This section aims to help you understand different learning styles and how to assess your own learning style as well as how to do a strengths, weaknesses, opportunities and threats (SWOT) analysis and set SMART(ER) goals. Understanding these things will help you to consolidate your learning in and out of the classroom and help you prepare for your assessments. There are some activities and case studies to help you consider how you might approach different scenarios or difficulties you could face.

All nursing courses are regulated, approved and monitored by the NMC, and theory and practice elements are equally valued. This is to ensure that nursing courses are designed to meet proficiencies and outcomes relevant to the course (NMC, 2023).

NMC

THE NMC SAYS

'Public safety is central to our standards. Students will be in contact with people throughout their education, and it's important that they learn in a safe and effective way'.

It is important to be aware that universities that run nursing courses do so in conjunction with many clinical practice partners and employers. This could include areas within the NHS as well as the private and voluntary sectors. These partnerships are vital to ensure that you are fully prepared when registering with the NMC.

NMC

THE NMC SAYS

'Approved education institutions (AEIs) are responsible for working with practice learning partners to manage the quality of their educational programmes.'

Attendance and engagement

Attendance and engagement are closely monitored, both in theory (at the university) and in practice placements. Your teaching on a nursing course is likely to be delivered in a combination of ways. You will likely attend the following:

- Lectures—often delivered in larger groups and will likely have a lecturer providing a presentation or information.
- Seminars—often facilitated in smaller groups, and these provide an opportunity for students to discuss topics in more detail and complete activities.
- Skills or simulation—often take place in a skills laboratory (a room set up to replicate a hospital ward or community setting), and students will have the opportunity to practice clinical and communication skills.
- Clinical practice learning—these will take place in clinical placement/ work-based learning areas. These may be within the NHS or the private/voluntary sector, where you will have the opportunity to link theory to practice, meaning that you will acquire new knowledge and skills as well as apply and consolidate the learning gained in the university environment.

(For further information on teaching delivery, see Chapter 2.)

The information given to you about the course modules/units will provide you with more information about how the content will be delivered.

Adult learning

It is important to be aware that studying a nursing course at university will be quite different from what you may have been used to at school or college. As adult learners, you will be responsible for your own success and will need to complete reading and activities outside of the taught sessions. This is often referred to as self-directed learning. Adult learning means that you have more freedom to learn in your own way and at a time that is right for you, but that does mean that you need to put in the time outside of the teaching sessions to continue your learning. Your lecturers and the module plans/module descriptors will be able to advise you about how much time you are expected to complete as self-directed learning as well as tasks that need to be completed. Self-directed study gives you as the student ownership for your development and is essential for succeeding in the nursing course.

Look at the module plans/descriptors for each of your first-semester modules. Find out how many hours are allocated for taught sessions and for self-directed learning.

How will you find protected time to meet these requirements? Make notes in the space below.

_____

_____

_____

_____

Hybrid learning

As we have mentioned, nursing courses are professional courses that are regulated by the NMC; therefore, it is likely that much of the taught content will be delivered on campus, face to face. However, some universities now adopt a hybrid approach to delivering nursing courses, to some extent.

Hybrid learning, also sometimes referred to as blended learning, combines face-to-face teaching sessions and online teaching sessions and/or self-directed or group activities. Using a hybrid approach has many benefits such as providing students with more flexibility, helping reduce travel and or childcare costs and providing students with more independence to adopt their own learning styles and take ownership of their learning. A hybrid course delivery strikes a balance in education, which many students prefer to traditional course delivery methods. However, students can also face challenges with hybrid learning. Before starting a nursing course that utilises a hybrid approach, you will need to ensure that you have access to a laptop/computer and sufficient internet access; these will be essential for accessing online sessions/activities. If you are concerned about this, seek support and guidance from your university lecturers as soon as possible. Some students can find online sessions isolating and lonely, as you are more disconnected from peers and university staff. However, this is less likely with a hybrid approach, as the online sessions are used in conjunction with face-to-face classroom teaching and used to complement the learning process. (Further information about online teaching and learning is in Chapter 2.)

SOCIAL MEDIA
@AmyPile4

'Engaging with online breakout groups is really important, being the chosen speaker for the breakout group takes you out of your comfort zone, it really builds up your confidence and increases your articulation'

TIP

When attending online sessions or activities, ensure that you have a quiet space to work with minimal distractions around you. You will often be required to turn on your laptop camera and or microphone in order to participate fully, so make sure these are working in advance.

Look at the course handbook and course plan and make sure that you understand how the university you are attending delivers the nursing course. Do they use a hybrid approach? If so, use the space below to think about any barriers you think you might face with this approach, and consider how you might overcome these.

_____

_____

_____

_____

SWOT analysis and SMART(ER) goals

SWOT analysis

When starting a nursing course at university, it is important to identify your strengths and weaknesses and to create learning goals. This is particularly important during your first year of studying, when you are receiving a large amount of information and you might be new to the concept of adult learning. SWOT analysis is a technique used to help identify your personal **strengths** and **weaknesses** and helps us to identify learning **opportunities** and minimise potential **threats**. It is important for us to understand these aspects of ourselves, so we can lean into the areas in which we excel at but also identify areas where we need to further develop (Fig. 1.1).

SMART(ER) goals

Once you have completed your SWOT analysis, it is important to set goals. Yes, your ultimate goal is likely to successfully complete the course and become a registered nurse; however, setting yourself smaller goals along the way can make it easier to focus and make your overall goal feel more achievable. We recommend that for each of your modules, you consider what your aims are for a particular module and create a plan for completing the assessment (See Chapter 6), including what resources you might need to help you achieve your goal.

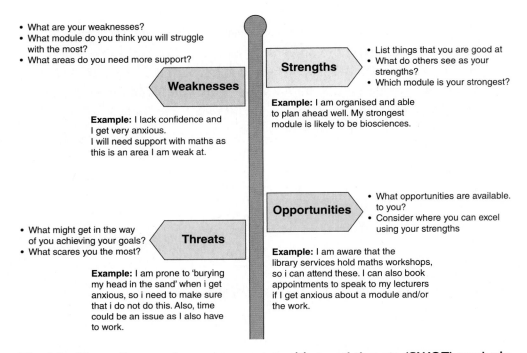

- What are your weaknesses?
- What module do you think you will struggle with the most?
- What areas do you need more support?

Weaknesses

Example: I lack confidence and I get very anxious.
I will need support with maths as this is an area I am weak at.

Strengths

- List things that you are good at
- What do others see as your strengths?
- Which module is your strongest?

Example: I am organised and able to plan ahead well. My strongest module is likely to be biosciences.

Opportunities

- What opportunities are available. to you?
- Consider where you can excel using your strengths

- What might get in the way of you achieving your goals?
- What scares you the most?

Threats

Example: I am prone to 'burying my head in the sand' when i get anxious, so i need to make sure that i do not do this. Also, time could be an issue as I also have to work.

Example: I am aware that the library services hold maths workshops, so i can attend these. I can also book appointments to speak to my lecturers if I get anxious about a module and/or the work.

Fig. 1.1   Strengths, weaknesses, opportunities and threats (SWOT) analysis.

When creating goals, it is advised that you use a SMART(ER) criteria. SMART(ER) is a mnemonic acronym which helps you consider a systematic approach to writing objectives (Fig. 1.2).

Complete a SMART(ER) goal for each of your modules and assessments.

What are your key goals from carrying out this activity?

How will you achieve them?

_____

_____

_____

_____

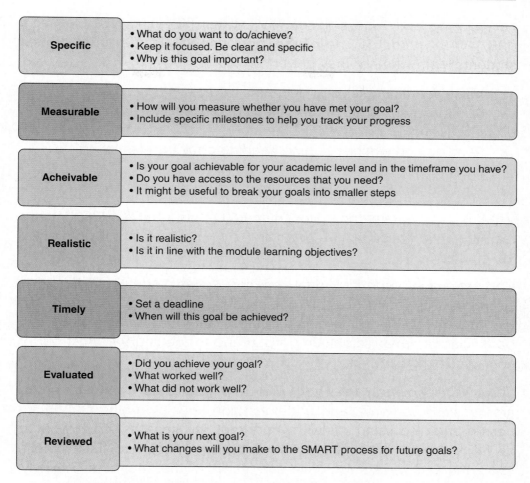

Specific	• What do you want to do/achieve? • Keep it focused. Be clear and specific • Why is this goal important?
Measurable	• How will you measure whether you have met your goal? • Include specific milestones to help you track your progress
Acheivable	• Is your goal achievable for your academic level and in the timeframe you have? • Do you have access to the resources that you need? • It might be useful to break your goals into smaller steps
Realistic	• Is it realistic? • Is it in line with the module learning objectives?
Timely	• Set a deadline • When will this goal be achieved?
Evaluated	• Did you achieve your goal? • What worked well? • What did not work well?
Reviewed	• What is your next goal? • What changes will you make to the SMART process for future goals?

Fig. 1.2   SMART(ER) criteria for systematic approach to writing objectives.

Learning styles

As well as recognising our strengths and weakness, it is important that as adult learners, we understand learning styles. There are many different learning styles which you will encounter during your nursing course. One way you can use learning styles is by trying different approaches so you have a 'toolbox' of methods to draw on, dependent on the task at hand. We all have our own preferred learning style depending on the subject matter and the learning environment. There are many ways of categorising and assessing learning styles; however, Neil Fleming's (1987) VARK model is one of the most popular. In the VARK model, students learn whether they prefer

- Visual learning (pictures, diagrams, videos, mind maps)
- Auditory learning (lectures, listening to speakers, music, peer discussions)
- Reading and writing learning (reading books or journal articles, creating lists)
- Kinaesthetic learning (hands-on activities, practical sessions)

VARK is one of many tools. Honey and Mumford (1986a: 1986b) offer a learning style questionnaire that can help you find out your preferred learning style(s).

Understanding your individual learning styles and identifying your strengths and weaknesses are not just beneficial for understanding the taught content during the nursing course; they can also be extremely beneficial for when completing group and for getting the most out of your clinical placements.

Throughout your studies, you will be expected to complete group activities/assessments, and understanding your strengths and weaknesses and discussing this with your group will help the group work to its full potential. When we acknowledge and embrace each other's strengths and weaknesses, we can lean into the strengths. Similarly, at the beginning of each placement you have, you will meet with a member of staff to discuss your learning objectives. This will be known as your practice supervisor or practice assessor. Discussing your learning style and your strengths and limitations will help the staff know how to best support you and which areas you may need to develop during your time with them.

NMC | THE NMC SAYS

8.1 'Respect the skills, expertise and contributions of your colleagues, referring matters to them when appropriate'.

CASE STUDY

Kai has just finished his A levels, and a hybrid curriculum is a new concept to him, as he is used to face-to-face classroom-based learning. Whilst Kia likes the flexibility of online sessions and activities, he struggles to engage with these sessions and is falling behind with his learning.

What would you suggest to Kia?

[Our suggestion] It is common to struggle to engage with online sessions at times, and some students do find themselves less motivated when it comes to online learning. It is important to fully participate with the session and interact with the content. Have your camera turned on, and if allowed, use your microphone to ask/answer questions, rather than using the chat box. Be sure to participate in any group activities; it is easy to sit back and not engage in this when online, but the more you participate, the more interesting you will find it, and in turn, you will learn more. It is important to be prepared for seminars; in doing so, you will increase your confidence and make it easier to engage and contribute. It might also be helpful to reflect on the learning process after the sessions to see what worked well for you and what didn't.

CASE STUDY

Natasha is a mature student and has not studied for many years. Natasha is a single mum and is finding it hard to complete the self-directed study and is feeling anxious about the assessments for each module.

What would you suggest to Natasha?

[Our suggestion] It is easy to become anxious and overwhelmed by the workload and the assessments; it's important to be organised and plan ahead. It may help Natasha if she created a SMART(ER) goal for each module. Many students also find it useful to create a planner for each module with clear objectives for each week for each

Continued

CASE STUDY—cont'd

module and to map out time to complete these. It is also important to remember to seek support from staff at the university if you are feeling overwhelmed. This could be the module leaders, personal tutor and also support services, such as the library or digital learning teams, who often provide support and advice around assessments. We will discuss the support available to students in more detail in the next section. Do not forget the importance of peers when it comes to support and motivation too. It might be helpful to start a study group with your peers or join an existing one and complete self-directed study or prepare for assessments together.

LOOKING AFTER YOUR WELL-BEING AND MAXIMISING THE SUPPORT TO THRIVE AT UNIVERSITY

Well-being, self-care and health

Through this chapter, we have recognised that starting at university and becoming a nursing student is exciting but can equally be challenging. So far, this chapter has discussed some of the practicalities around starting a nursing course at university. It has given you some ideas of what you can do to be prepared and organised to maximise your experience and learning potential both within the university and when on placement.

Looking after your health and well-being is very important, and as a society, we are much more aware of the importance of maintaining and protecting our own health. When we discuss health and well-being, we often think about our physical health, but this also includes other areas such as our happiness, emotional well-being and mental health.

This section of the chapter will look at some wider aspects of health and well-being, as well as considering some of the support that might be available to you on your nursing course at university.

Well-being

Well-being looks at all aspects of a person, particularly focusing on how someone feels and how this impacts how they function and reach their full potential. The health and well-being of those working in nursing now are considered not only important but an absolute essential priority (Blake and Stacey, 2022).

'If we feel good, we are much more likely to feel more positive and be more successful. If we feel unwell, low in mood or stressed we may not be working to our full potential'.

Phill Hoddinott and Jennifer Hanley, senior lecturers in nursing

'Working in healthcare (as a student or professional) is really rewarding but can be incredibly draining mentally and emotionally. Making a proactive effort in protecting your mental health and well-being, as I have experienced this year, is so important not only for yourself but also for your development as a nurse. It's great caring for others, but you have to care for yourself too'!

Ella Isaac, student nurse, London South Bank University

As a nursing student undertaking a placement, you will come across patients and service users who might have a distressing, critical or chronic illness/ injury and are vulnerable. You may have to support their families or other members of healthcare staff through difficult times. It is important that we are physically and mentally fit enough ourselves to provide good-quality nursing care and support all those we look after and work with. Effectively looking after our own health and managing our own self-care is a practical way to ensure that we are positively managing our own well-being.

NMC

THE NMC SAYS

20.9 'Maintain the level of health you need to carry out your professional role'.

Self-care

Self-care is an important tool to maintain your well-being. Self-care is about the management of yourself and making the time to do things that help you live well, feel good and improve all aspects of your health (Blake and Stacey, 2022). Self-care can focus on living a healthier life such as exercising and cooking homemade healthy food. Other areas could include maintaining and building friendship groups, spending time with your family or going on holiday.

Self-care does not have to be big and expensive; it can be based around simple things that you enjoy doing such as reading a book, going to the cinema or making sure you can attend spiritual or social activities.

TIP

There are many podcasts around maintaining your well-being and promoting self-care such as practising mindfulness or meditation. Take a look at your preferred podcast provider; many are free.

Life balance

This chapter has previously discussed the importance of effectively organising yourself and your studies. It is equally important to ensure that other areas of your life are equally as well organised and not neglected. All humans are multidimensional, and we have many different roles and identities; being a nursing student is just one part of you and one that you need to adapt to. Making sure that you have room in your life to relax, enjoy some free time and have time to maintain friendships/do hobbies are all important parts of enhancing and maintaining your well-being through self-care.

When planning your time around your lectures, coursework/exam deadlines and placement dates, be sure to factor in time for you to prioritise other areas of your life. Maybe you have a family and need to focus on spending some quality time with your partner or children? Do you need to do part-time work to support yourself financially?

TIP

Why not ask the SU what clubs and societies they run? This is a good way of finding or maintaining a hobby, meeting new people and contributing to the university community.

Physical health

Making sure we are physically fit and well is an important part of our well-being. As a nursing student, you might have moved away from home, so it's important that you register with a local GP and dentist. This will ensure that you can get medical and dental treatment easily and locally to where you are living and studying. Healthcare is about keeping well and not just about managing illness, so being able to access local healthcare services is important (Blake and Stacey, 2022). Knowledge about healthcare in your local community is important, this includes knowing where your local pharmacy, contraception and sexual health services are based.

The 111 NHS telephone service can often give expert nonurgent advice. If there is a medical emergency or someone needs immediate medical help or attention, always call 999 or visit the nearest accident and emergency (A&E) department.

TIP

Your university will often have details or will be able to signpost students to local healthcare services; some might even have these services on campus. Find out and register with a GP or dentist as soon as possible.

Mental health

Mental health and well-being go hand in hand, and it is important that we value positive mental health as well as understand what can impact our mental health and who can help during times of difficulty.

Maintaining well-being and managing self-care and life balance are all important tools that can positively impact your quality of life and have a direct impact on your mental health and well-being. Activities such as mindfulness, reflection and peer support are all tools that can help us deal with everyday life as well as some of the more complex situations around being a nursing student.

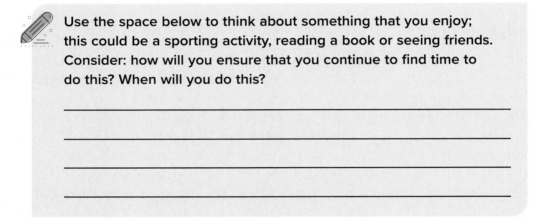

Use the space below to think about something that you enjoy; this could be a sporting activity, reading a book or seeing friends. Consider: how will you ensure that you continue to find time to do this? When will you do this?

Sometimes everyone feels low, upset or stressed; this is normal, but it is important to recognise the signs and symptoms of poor or deteriorating mental health and know where you can get help. The section below around support on your nursing course can guide you to the support structures within your university and peer support. If you have any mental health concerns, you should discuss them with your GP or other health-care professional. In case of an emergency, the NHS telephone services can often give expert advice, and always call 999 or visit the nearest A&E department if you have immediate mental health issues or concerns.

There are many telephone, web and social media services that can offer mental health and emotional support. Organisations such as The

Samaritans are open 24 hours a day, 365 days of the year, and can offer help and support during a metal health crisis. There are also student-focused support services that can be accessed free of charge. These include Student Minds (https://www.studentminds.org.uk/) and Student Space (https://studentspace.org.uk/).

Support available to you on your nursing course at university

While we hope that your journey to becoming a registered nurse is a positive one, it is not uncommon to come across challenging times throughout the duration. Nursing courses are extremely rewarding, but completing a professional qualification can be tough at times, and this can be for a variety of reasons, which could include personal and academic-related issues.

The previous section explained the importance of looking after your health and well-being, and there will be a wide range of support that your university can offer to help you succeed. It is important to be aware of the support that is available to you should you experience any struggles or difficulties. At the beginning of the course, you should make note of the support services offered by your university.

Although at the time you might think that you won't need it, it is better to have this information to hand should you find yourself struggling one day; this way you can access help quickly.

Course information

Lots of information will be given to you during your induction to the university and nursing course. Section 1 of this chapter has given you some helpful activities around making sure you are as organised as you can be at the start of your course. The student handbook or course guide will provide you with further information about the support services available at your specific university, so ensure that you read this and keep this handy so you can refer to it when you are unsure of something or need signposting to help and support.

TIP

Remember, it is important to ask for help and support when you need it. Staff at the university want to help you and want you to reach your full potential in your studies; however, to do so, you need to tell them when you need help.

Now let's consider some people and roles in the university who will be able to support, guide and help you throughout your nursing course.

- **Personal tutor**—At the start of your nursing course, you will be allocated a personal tutor for the duration of the course. Usually, your personal tutor will be a member of the academic team in the department of your field of nursing, and their role is to support you in achieving your academic and practice-related learning outcomes. Usually, your personal tutor will be your first line of contact should you have any queries or concerns during your time on the course. If you are an apprentice, this role may be called something different, or indeed, you may have additional roles aimed at supporting you with the apprenticeship requirements and employer communication.
- **Course leader/course director**—Course leaders or course directors are responsible for the day-to-day delivery and coordination of your course. Their role is to ensure the nursing courses are delivered as efficiently as possible.
- **Cohort leads or year leads**—Most universities will have a person allocated as either a cohort lead or year lead. The role of these individuals is to focus more on group and professional issues raised by the cohort, as well as keeping the cohort informed of developments within the university and in professional practice.
- **Link lecturer**—A link lecturer is a member of staff responsible for liaising with the university partner trusts. They liaise with these areas on a regular basis and are responsible for supporting nursing students whilst out on clinical placements.
- **Academic assessor**—In the Standards for Student Supervision and Assessment (NMC, 2018b), all students will be allocated an

academic assessor whilst out on clinical placement. The academic assessor will work with a nominated practice assessor (who is based in the clinical area) to make a recommendation for student progression. This is to ensure safe and effective learning.

Who are the people who can support you throughout the duration of your nursing programme?

Make a note of their name, title and contact details in space below.

_____

_____

_____

_____

Now let's take a look at what teams and services in many universities are available to provide you with support.

Student services

Most universities have a department which is often referred to as student services (the name might differ slightly at different establishments). The aim of the student services team is to assist all students to fulfil their full potential while studying. The student services team will be able to offer support and advice to students, so do not hesitate to contact them should you have any questions or concerns. Student services will be your first point of contact should you have any questions or need support about the following:

- Student finance/fees
- Accommodation
- Hardship funds
- Mental health and well-being support
- Assessing counselling

Student mental health and well-being service

The student mental health and well-being service offers advice and support to students who are experiencing personal difficulties. This service will be free and confidential. You can seek support from the team for matters directly relating to the course, but you can also seek support for personal matters not related to the course. A mental health and well-being adviser will discuss your concerns and difficulties with you as well as the impact this might be having on your studies. They will help you to think about what might help improve the situation, and this will probably include creating a support plan with you. Support will often be available to you in a variety of different methods; this might include counselling/support face to face, virtually or over the phone.

Disability support services

The Equality Act (2010) states that all higher education providers must ensure that students with disabilities are not treated less favourably than other students, and they have a duty to make reasonable adjustments. The university disability support team is a dedicated service for students who have a disability that could be a physical medical condition, mental health condition, learning difficulties or neurodiversity. The disability support team can offer a range of services and support to those who register with them. It is important to note that students do not have to register with the disability team; however, you may be entitled to additional support which could include equipment, additional time for assessments or financial support through the Disabled Students Allowance to help you with your studies, which would only be available to you if you register with the team. More information can be found at https://www.gov.uk/disabled-students-allowance-dsa. Registering with the team will enable them to provide you with an individual plan aimed at supporting you with your specific needs.

If you have never been assessed for learning differences, which could include dyslexia, dyspraxia, dyscalculia and attention deficit hyperactivity disorder, but feel like you would benefit from this, then the Disability Support service can support you with this. (Refer to Chapter 11.)

Spiritual support/chaplaincy

All universities have a multifaith chaplaincy which students can access for pastoral support throughout the course. A chaplain is a leader in their own faith but also works closely with other faiths. You will be able to talk in confidence to the chaplains about matters of religion or any other worries or issues you may have. They are here to help students and staff of all faiths or none.

Peer support

Peer support will be essential during your time studying on a nursing course. Whilst, as we have discussed earlier, there are numerous individuals and services that are available to support and advise you throughout your studies, the support your peers can provide will be invaluable. Sometimes when we are experiencing challenges or lacking motivation, we feel more comfortable talking to our friends about it.

Support from social media

Social media can also be a great supportive tool. Twitter can be a valuable resource for networking and obtaining advice. If you experience a difficult situation whilst at university or in clinical practice, it can be useful to discuss this with peers far and wide via Twitter. Be sure to use social media and social networking sites responsibly and in line with the NMC guidance on using social media responsibly (NMC, 2015).

CASE STUDY

Akrem is finding the academic work at university challenging. They complete all of the presession reading and have attended every lecture, but they are finding it difficult to recall information, and they find that their notes do not help, as they do not make any sense after the session. Akrem struggled with this at school and just thinks this is because they are not very good at academic work.

Continued

CASE STUDY—cont'd

What would you suggest to Akrem?

[Our suggestion] It is estimated that 10% of the UK population may have a learning difference such as dyslexia. This is often identified during university study, and difficulties that a person may have encountered at school are explained. Akrem could speak to his personal tutor about the problems they are facing as well as making some enquires about the university disability support services, who can often arrange assessment and, where required, access to wider support such as reasonable adjustments to help Akrem with their learning both at university and whilst on clinical placements.

CASE STUDY

Sukki has just started her first placement and is finding the experience overwhelming. She often goes home feeling sad when she witnesses people who are extremely unwell, and when a patient died when she was on shift, she had to go and sit in the staff room and could not stop crying.

What would you suggest to Sukki?

[Our suggestion] Practice learning can be really challenging, as it's an unpredictable learning environment. Supporting and nursing sick people and their families can often be highly stressful and emotional. Sukki could speak to someone on her placement such as her practice assessor, so they can support and help her to process this. Sukki's link lecturer is also a good person to talk to about issues around her clinical placements.

It is important that Sukki remembers that even when she is on placement, she is still a student at her university, and keeping in

CASE STUDY—cont'd

touch with her personal tutor is also a good way to get support. Sometimes everyone needs a little extra support, and talking to an impartial person could help Sukki to understand her thoughts and feelings by accessing student mental health and well-being and spiritual support/chaplaincy services.

Finally, Sukki should think about her plan that she has made to look after her well-being and use her support network such as her peers, family and friends.

CONCLUSION

Starting a nursing course at university is a positive life-changing experience. Settling into university life is exciting but also comes with some challenges, particularly adjusting to adult higher education ways of learning.

This chapter has explored some areas to help you to prepare and settle into your first year on your nursing course at university. It has made reference to adult learning styles and identified some support and well-being services that can help you thrive but also survive, particularly during challenging times. You have been invited to further consider supporting your own success through developing a plan to thrive, survive and succeed during your first year and help you to prepare for the remainder of your nursing course.

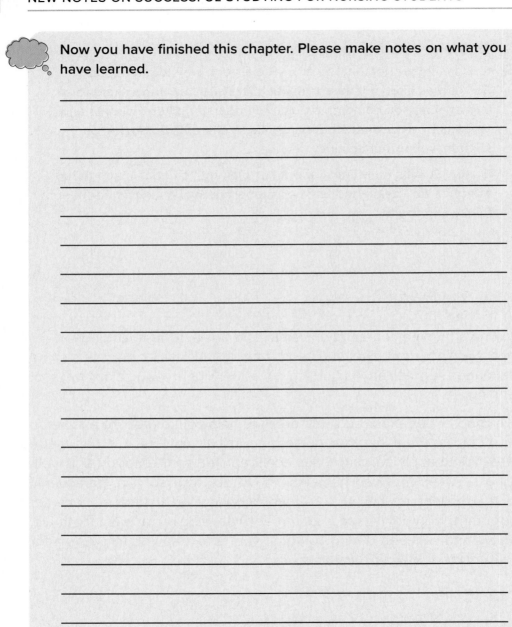

Now you have finished this chapter. Please make notes on what you have learned.

REFERENCES

Atkinson, S. (2022) Imposter syndrome can occur at any stage of the nursing journey, Available at: https://www.nursingtimes.net/students/imposter-syndrome-can-occur-at-any-stage-of-the-nursing-journey-07-11-2022/. (Accessed: 20/06/23).

Blake, H. and Stacey, G. (2022) Health and Well-being at Work for Nurses and Midwives, 1 ed., London: Elsevier Health Sciences.

Equality Act (2010) Available at https://www.legislation.gov.uk/ukpga/2010/15/contents. Accessed 30.1.24

Flemming, N (1987) Introduction to VARK for better learning. Available at https://vark-learn.com/introduction-to-vark/. Accessed on 30.1.2024

Honey, P. and Mumford, A. (1986a) *The Manual of Learning Styles*, Peter Honey Associates.

Honey, P. and Mumford, A. (1986b) *Learning Styles Questionnaire*, Peter Honey Publications Ltd.

Nursing and Midwifery Council (NMC), (2015) Guidance on using social media responsibly, Available at: https://www.nmc.org.uk/globalassets/sitedocuments/nmc-publications/social-media-guidance.pdf (Accessed: 20/06/23).

Nursing and Midwifery Council (NMC), (2018b). Standards for student supervision and assessment. Available at: https://www.nmc.org.uk/globalassets/sitedocuments/standards/2023-pre-reg-standards/new-vi/standards-for-student-supervision-and-assessment.pdf (Accessed: 20/06/23).

Nursing and Midwifery Council (NMC), (2019). Guidance on health and character. London: NMC. Available at: https://www.nmc.org.uk/globalassets/sitedocuments/nmc-publications/guidance-on-health-and-character/ (Accessed: 20/06/23).

Nursing and Midwifery Council (NMC), (2023). Standards framework for nursing and midwifery education. Available at: https://www.nmc.org.uk/globalassets/sitedocuments/standards/2023-pre-reg-standards/new-vi/standards-framework-for-nursing-and-midwifery-education.pdf (Accessed: 20/06/23).

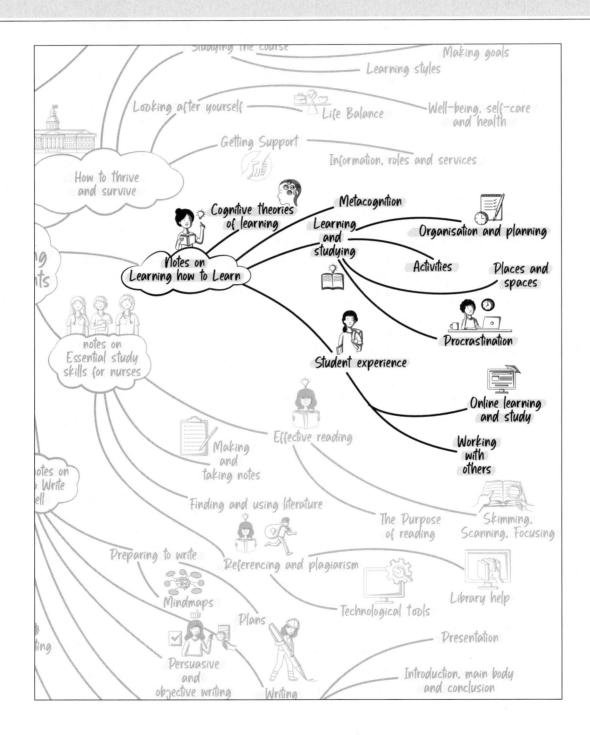

Studying the course

Making goals

Learning styles

Looking after yourself — Life Balance — Well-being, self-care and health

Getting Support

Information, roles and services

How to thrive and survive

Cognitive theories of learning — Metacognition

Learning and studying — Organisation and planning

Notes on Learning how to Learn

Activities

Places and spaces

Procrastination

Student experience

Online learning and study

Working with others

notes on Essential study skills for nurses

Making and taking notes

Effective reading

Finding and using literature

The Purpose of reading

Skimming, Scanning, Focusing

Referencing and plagiarism

Library help

Preparing to write

otes on o Write ell

Mindmaps

Technological tools

Plans

Presentation

Persuasive and objective writing

Writing

Introduction, main body and conclusion

NOTES ON LEARNING HOW TO LEARN

Fi Croucher (She/her) ∎ **Andrea Cockett** ∎
Jennie Brady (She/her)

INTRODUCTION

Understanding how we all learn and developing good study skills can make a big difference in your experience in your nursing programme. It is important that you develop approaches to studying that work for you. In this chapter, you are going to be introduced to some of the theory underpinning learning, how this can influence your ability to study effectively and how you can organise yourself to optimise your studying. Understanding how we learn will also help you to develop the role of the teacher. This is a key Nursing and Midwifery Council (NMC) (2018a) proficiency, and it is important that by the end of your programme, you have developed the skills and knowledge that will enable you to teach and support others with their learning in the clinical practice environment. In addition, in this chapter, we will also explore strategies to effectively manage procrastination, navigate the realm of blended or online learning and recognise the significance of collaborating harmoniously with peers and colleagues.

NMC

THE NMC SAYS

5.8: 'Support and supervise students in the delivery of nursing care, promoting reflection and providing constructive feedback, and evaluating and documenting their performance'.

Annex A: 4.1: 'Demonstrate effective supervision, teaching and performance appraisal'.

There are lots of different theories presented in the literature about how people learn, and in the first part of this chapter, you are going to be introduced to one theory that has been influential on our current understanding of learning. It has been included, as it will be useful to you in relation to developing your own understanding of learning to inform your study skills. There is not one universally accepted theory of learning, and it is important to understand this and to recognise that we will all learn different concepts in different ways throughout our life. In older publications, you might see references to something called learning styles. This idea suggests that we all have a fixed learning style which is our preferred way to learn; however, we now know that this is not the case, and we can all learn to learn in different ways (Hughes, 2020) (See Chapter 1).

One educational psychological theory that can be universally applied is that of cognitive theories of learning and, particularly, metacognition. Penn (2020) refers to it as the key to successful studying, so it is a useful theory to develop your understanding of.

COGNITIVE THEORIES OF LEARNING AND METACOGNITION

Cognition relates to the mental processes involved in thinking, perceiving, problem-solving and remembering (Rutherford-Hemming, 2012). Cognitive learning theories focus on the mechanisms that are used by the brain to process, store and retrieve information. A key component of cognitive learning is the internal mental processes that we undertake to actively increase our knowledge and skills. An important component of this is being able to identify our current level of knowledge and the gaps we need to fill to enhance and develop it. There is a strong focus on active learning processes in cognitive theories (Allen, 2007). What this means is that to learn successfully, you need to be an active participant in the learning activities that you will undertake as part of your course. What this means will be discussed a little later in this chapter.

Metacognition is a key component of cognitive learning theories. Metacognition is thinking about how we think. It is the processes that we can use to plan, monitor and assess our own understanding and performance. This is important because we often overestimate our own competence and abilities, which can lead to less effective learning (Kruger and Dunning, 1999; Penn, 2020).

Metacognitive ability is the skill of being able to monitor and evaluate your own current level of attainment and therefore be able to identify what you need to learn (Penn, 2020). Linked to metacognitive ability is our understanding of how we can retain and use information effectively. Again, the literature suggests that most of us overestimate our ability to retain and apply information (Koriat and Bjork, 2005). This can then lead us to use ineffective study methods, as we believe by, for example, rereading texts, we have retained and understood the information (Hughes, 2020). The evidence would suggest that the most effective way for us to understand how much knowledge we have retained is to test ourselves (Penn, 2020).

Understanding the concept of metacognition can help us to use more productive study methods that allow us to:

- Understand where the gaps in our knowledge are
- Identify what information we have retained and are able to apply to different problems/situations
- Identify areas of knowledge that we need to spend more time focusing our study efforts on

So, what does this actually mean for you as a nursing student? What this means is that you need to use study methods that are *active* and not *passive*. Examples of passive learning activities would be:

- Sitting in a lecture and not taking notes
- Reading an article or book chapter and not taking notes from it (evidence shows that highlighting texts you are reading is not effective! [Penn, 2020])
- Not participating in group discussions, either online or in person

What we know from cognitive learning theories is that there are some key things you can do that will help you retain and then recall information in order to develop your knowledge and skills. These include:

- Taking notes in lectures and seminars and from books and articles, preferably by hand, as this has been shown to be effective

- Organising yourself to optimise your studying
- Testing yourself to ensure you can recall knowledge

TIP

Think about what activities you normally undertake when listening to lectures or reading texts. Try to incorporate more active methods into these activities so you are an active, not a passive, learner.

LEARNING AND STUDYING

Learning is all about developing your knowledge and skills. It's not limited to a specific place or time. The experiences that you have in a classroom, online, while reading a book or through placement all contribute to the development of your knowledge and skills. When we learn, we are building our knowledge and skills all the time; you should see learning as a continuous process in which you develop and refine your knowledge and skills with every learning activity you undertake or experience you have. Studying is a specific process within the broader concept of learning. It's the focused act of developing knowledge by searching for information, reviewing materials and practising what you've learned. When you're studying, you're actively seeking out information, whether it's from textbooks, journals, online resources or discussions with your peers or lecturers. It's all about diving into the content, understanding it and making connections. Studying is like putting together puzzle pieces to see the bigger picture.

The next section of this chapter will explore some of these ideas to help you to make the most of the study time that you have available to learn.

Organising yourself for successful studying

In order to be successful on your course, you will need to develop strong organisational study skills. This will involve you undertaking different learning activities, managing your assessments and balancing this alongside clinical placements. When you start university, it is easy to throw yourself into your studies and other activities with a huge amount of enthusiasm, but we know that these early intense few weeks are often not sustainable in the longer term and can lead to you losing your motivation. As outlined in Chapter 1, it is important for your success and well-being that you adopt good study practices that will allow you to achieve a balanced approach to your programme, get the most from the opportunities that university offers and be successful. This section provides information for you on how you can do this.

Types of learning activities

At university, you will experience lots of different learning activities. Some of these will be fully directed by staff (as introduced to you in Chapter 1), for example, lectures, whilst others will require you to work independently or in groups. There will be opportunities for discussion, reflection and teamwork. Table 2.1 identifies some of the different types of learning activities you may encounter:

Whatever learning activity you are undertaking, it is important that you:

- Identify the value of the activity to your personal learning
- Engage fully with the learning activity
- Undertake any preparatory activities
- Reflect on the activity and identify your learning and any further activities you need to undertake to enhance it (Cottrell, 2019)

This will then enable you to make the most of the activity and optimise your learning from it.

Organising and planning your learning

As a nursing student, you will have lots of demands on your time, so it is important to think about how you can manage your time productively and maintain both your enthusiasm and well-being. Hughes (2020) suggests that there are three factors we need to consider that can impact on our well-being that relate to learning:

1. **Your psychological engagement with learning**: Are you focused on grades or on learning, do you have emotional engagement with the topics you are studying and how motivated are you?
2. **Your level of skill and feelings of mastery**: How competent you feel about an academic task will influence your feelings about undertaking it.

TABLE 2.1 TYPES OF LEARNING ACTIVITIES

Lecture

Lectures are used to provide you with an overview of a topic. They can either be in person, live online or pre-recorded. You should view them as an introduction to a topic rather than being a source of all the information that you may need. Lectures should be viewed as a starting point from which you can then further explore the topic, either in a linked seminar or in directed learning activities. It is important to ensure you have completed any introductory activities required before engaging with a lecture and make sure that you are attentive throughout.

Directed reading

Reading is a fundamental skill that you need to develop in order to be successful at university. Directed readings will be core texts that you need to become familiar with about a particular topic. They could be book chapters, journal articles or policies.

Group work

This is often used in seminars to provide you with opportunities for discussion in smaller groups in order to develop your knowledge and understanding.

Simulation

This is an immersive experience in which you will role play clinical situations and combine your theoretical knowledge with your clinical skills.

Mandatory training

This is training that all students on nursing programmes must complete and includes things like basic life support, first aid and moving and handling training.

Seminar

Seminars are used for discussion, clarification and to build on the knowledge discussed in a lecture. Seminars are your opportunity to ask any questions you may have, voice your thoughts on a topic and develop your knowledge further. Seminars often have activities or readings identified that you need to complete prior to attending and we know that the more you participate the more you will gain.

E learning

Interactive e-learning has become a key feature of many programmes. E learning activities are designed to be self-paced and provide you with interactive opportunities to learn more about a topic. It may be used for preparatory activities or to develop your knowledge of a topic.

Clinical skills teaching

This is a core component of all nursing programmes and provides an opportunity to rehearse and develop competency in clinical skills before undertaking them in the practice environment.

Interactive online activities

Lots of programmes now use interactive online activities such as Padlet and Jamboard that allow you to interact with academic staff and other students inside and outside of scheduled teaching time. You will also use virtual learning environments such as Blackboard, Moodle or Canvas. These are used to support your learning activities and help you to organise and sequence your study time.

3. **Your grades and the value you attach to achievement**: When we get the grades we are hoping for, that can improve our motivation and attitudes towards learning, but lower grades can also be used as motivators, so how you view your grades can influence your learning and well-being.

These three factors can all be managed by adopting a structured approach to study but also by recognising that there will be times when our motivation is lower, and we need to allow ourselves some time to reflect and pause on our study activities.

Students who take an organised approach to their study time will often have greater satisfaction with their outputs and efforts, as they do not feel under as much pressure when completing tasks, in particular, assessments (Cottrell, 2019). For nursing students, this can be particularly important, as you are balancing placements and university study.

 TIP

Think about what motivates you. Are you motivated by grades or by learning activities? Identifying what motivates you can help you to find motivation when it is lacking.

Study place and space

A key thing that often gets overlooked by students is the importance of finding the most suitable place to study. Everyone is different, and you may need to test what works for you. Some students prefer to use a personalised space, other study spaces such as university libraries or computer workrooms and some in more public spaces such as cafes. If you find that you lose concentration when staying in one place for a long period of time, you may need to have a regular change of scenery to be productive. For studying at home or in your university accommodation, ensure you separate your studying space from your relaxing space and that it is free from clutter and distractions. University study spaces may be busier at certain times of the day or week; knowing these will help you to choose the most conducive times for you to access them. Some universities have useful systems or apps to check real-time availability of seats in study spaces or even book them; make sure you benefit from using these. If you like to study in public spaces such as a cafe, choose somewhere local so you do not waste too much time travelling, ensure it has a reliable internet connection and find a small table in the corner away from the door and ordering counter.

It is important to recognise what your own organisational skills are and whether you need to spend some time at the beginning of each year, semester or term, outlining what learning activities and academic work have to be completed and when. You can use an online calendar accessible on your phone, tablet or computer; https://www.mystudylife.com/ and https://istudentpro.com/ are possible options. You can also easily create a planner or calendar using free downloadable templates, or you can purchase one. There are some great options at https://www.thehappystudentcompany.com/ and https://passionplanner.com/ (*please note these are recommendations only; we do not endorse any particular app or product*).

Time block/box all the activities you need to do to prepare for and complete each assessment; research shows this is more effective than to-do lists for work or studying (Rogers et al., 2015; Wu and Xie, 2018). You can use the suggested workload hours for each assessment in your module or unit scheme or handbook to help you. Further tips that can help you to be more organised are outlined as follows.

TIP

Organisation (Cottrell, 2019; Hughes, 2020)

STUDY STRATEGIES AND MINDSETS

- I think about my overall approach to my course
- I think about how I am going to achieve my best
- I am focused on continuous improvement
- I have a plan for each assessment task that I need to do
- I am an active learner and fully engaged with my course
- I understand how I can maximise my own learning
- I am reflective, so I learn from setbacks and activities that go well
- I don't give up when things are challenging
- I try to maintain my motivation

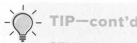

TIP—cont'd

STUDY SPACE

- I have a dedicated space that I use for study
- My space is organised, quiet and free of distractions
- I store all my materials in one place so I can access them easily
- My space supports my well-being when studying by having a suitable physical environment
- I have identified spaces on campus that I can also use to study in

RESOURCES

- I keep all of my resources labelled, well organised and easy to find; this includes my paper and electronic resources
- I have a good understanding of the learning technologies I need to use
- I use technology to help make organisation easier by optimising things like reminders and other tools available to me

PLANNING AND PREPARATION

- I ensure that I have all of the resources that I need for each module/course at the start of the module/course
- I plan well in advance for assessment tasks
- I organise my weekly schedule, so I plan what academic tasks I need to undertake each week/day
- I use a checklist system to keep track of my progress with tasks/assessments
- I ensure I am aware of the learning activities for each module and the assessment requirements
- I ensure that I keep track of all communications from the university/placements

LOOKING AFTER MY WELL-BEING

- I ensure I plan a balanced week and do not spend too much time studying
- I ensure that I am aware of where I can access support if I need it, both academic and pastoral
- I plan my weekly menu so that I am well nourished
- I plan to spend times with friends/family in the week
- I plan activities that I enjoy into my week

Reading and note-taking

Two key skills that can support your studying are effective reading and note-taking. Both of these skills are discussed in detail in Chapter 3 but are outlined briefly as follows.

Effective reading

Reading is crucial for effective learning activities, especially when preparing for assessments. To support your reading, be selective and consider the reading list provided by each module/course (Cottrell, 2019). A balanced approach is essential, considering the length of the assessment, topics covered and the number of resources needed for each section. Beware of overreading, which can lead to procrastination and unfocused writing (Hughes, 2020). Collecting resources actively is essential, as just reading and rereading a resource do not improve our understanding. To use sources effectively, we need to develop a deep understanding of them and use the knowledge gained to support our writing. Penn (2020) suggests an effective reading strategy: read, recite and review. This involves:

- **Reading** with purpose, identifying what we want to learn from the resource,
- **Reciting** everything we have read, and
- **Reviewing** by comparing notes with the resource and correcting any errors. By focusing on these strategies, you can develop a deep understanding of the material and use it to support your writing.

SOCIAL MEDIA
Ian@NTF_Ian

'Think about the quality of your reading. If you aren't reading high quality stuff it will massively impact on your writing. Always think about how this impacts on any practice/patient care. Why is something done that way is the key to critical analysis!'

This approach links to note-taking, which is discussed next, and incorporates testing, which is a key skill technique.

Effective note-taking

Effective note-taking is crucial for supporting learning activities and improving performance in assessments. It is not limited to lectures or face-to-face teaching but can also be used when reading or listening to online materials. Active participation in learning activities is essential, as memory does not function like a camera, and we reconstruct memories (Penn, 2020). Research suggests that active note-taking can improve assessment performance (Morehead et al., 2019), so it is a useful skill to develop. Research suggests that taking notes by hand is more effective than digitally (Morehead et al., 2019), and using a structured system can enhance the usefulness of your notes (Cottrell, 2019). In addition, annotating sources has not been shown to be particularly effective, so step away from the highlighters! (Penn, 2020). Some suggestions for structured notetaking systems are set out in Table 2.2.

One significant factor that can hinder our studying is procrastination, so developing an understanding of why we procrastinate and how we can manage it can be a great way of managing your time more effectively.

TABLE 2.2 TYPES OF NOTE-TAKING SYSTEMS

System	Structured note-taking systems
Cornell note-taking system	The Cornell note-taking system is a structured approach that can be used for taking notes from any source and provides you with a one-page summary of a learning activity.
Linear note-taking	Linear notes are note-taking as you listen to a lecture or read a source and are in chronological order.
Pattern notes	Pattern notes are more visual than Cornell or linear notes and comprise a diagram with the central idea in the middle and the information arranged diagrammatically around it.

Procrastination

We all have the capacity to procrastinate and lack motivation to study at times. It is important to recognise when we are doing this and for you to understand the triggers to your own procrastination. Procrastination can be related to our own feelings of self-efficacy, and one way of managing this is to be intentional (Penn, 2020). What this means is setting out clearly what we are going to do and when. For example, you could decide that you are going to undertake three 30-minute blocks of reading in a morning, so you would tell yourself, 'If I get out my journal articles, then I will read them'. This then provides a means of you setting out a goal and then measuring if you achieve it (Penn, 2020). Another useful strategy is to provide yourself with rewards for undertaking academic tasks, so, 'If I finish my three 30-minute reading blocks, I will have a break and go on social media for 10 minutes'. As discussed, managing distractions can be an important consideration in enabling us to undertake academic tasks in a timely and effective manner (Hughes, 2020). This could include using technology to limit your access to social media whilst you are studying (Penn, 2020).

There are some strategies for breaking a procrastination cycle that have been found to be useful. One is the Pomodoro technique (Cirillo, 2013). In this technique, you follow the following steps in Fig. 2.1:

This technique has been shown to work, as it can stop us from 'multitasking'. We know that people often look at lots of sources of information when they are using digital devices to study (Judd, 2015), that is, swapping between

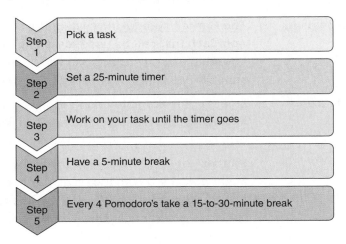

Step 1   Pick a task

Step 2   Set a 25-minute timer

Step 3   Work on your task until the timer goes

Step 4   Have a 5-minute break

Step 5   Every 4 Pomodoro's take a 15-to-30-minute break

Fig. 2.1   **The stages of the Pomodoro technique.**

study- and non-study-related activities when they are supposed to be focusing on studying. The Pomodoro technique can provide a focused way of managing these distractions by providing a learning environment in which distractions are minimised. This can increase your productivity and, if you are procrastinating, give you a kick start into a learning activity. This can be particularly important, as many nursing programmes are adopting blended learning approaches, which combine face-to-face and online activities. The next section of the chapter will discuss how you can study effectively online.

STUDENT EXPERIENCE

In this section, we'll explore insights from a nursing student on thoughts and feelings about starting a course of study and making online learning successful. This narrative aims to highlight the student's queries, identify the various types of support they received and provide some valuable tips for those of you on the same journey.

Please remember, as we move through this next section:

- How you are feeling or what you are worrying about is absolutely normal and to be expected
- You won't be the only student thinking and feeling like you do
- You are not on your own.

Receiving support whilst learning is really important because this enables students to get as much out of their education as possible. The updated NMC (2023) standards for pre-registration nursing programmes have been developed to better support students in achieving their required standards and proficiencies, and the structure has been developed to follow the student journey. These standards identify the expectation that learning support and supervision will be available and will support the delivery of safe and effective learning experiences (NMC, 2023).

Making online study work for you

A big part of making online study work for you is the need to have a degree of motivation, which can often be one of the main challenges. Al-Osaimi and Fawaz (2022) recognise motivation as an important driving force for academic success; it leads to increased engagement in learning activities and, therefore, an increased likelihood of achieving learning goals (Rafii et al., 2019).

To help you stay motivated to learn and produce academic work, seek useful connection with various members of the academic team, such as supervisors and module and programme leaders. Engaging in frequent learning conversations when studying remotely helps combat feelings of isolation and provides vital support. Learning conversations identify what is expected of you and help you recognise your strengths and weaknesses in relation to the learning activity or assessment task you are working on. They help you acutely focus on what is required and not what you think is required. These conversations should support open and honest discussion, allowing you to identify areas of achievement, skills that need further development as well as aspects of your work that need improvement.

As a first year, was the thought of online study worrying? If so, why?

CASE STUDY

Freddie is a first-year Adult Nursing Student who joins a group of students from different backgrounds and ages to share their fears and challenges about online learning. Some of them have studied recently, while others have taken a long break from education. They also have different levels of IT skills, ranging from confident to nervous. Freddie belongs to the latter group and feels very anxious about online study. The group decides to seek help from the University's academic skills support team to improve their IT skills. They also work together to learn how to use the various online platforms, explore their features, and find out their strengths and weaknesses as a group. Freddie shows initiative by attending some of the IT sessions. He also interacts regularly with his peers and takes part in the learning activities. As a result, he starts to feel more comfortable and confident in the online learning environment. He overcomes his initial fears and gains more trust in his ability to handle online studies.

It needs to be identified that there is a difference between online learning as a sole way to learn and it being part of a blended delivery. Blended delivery came to the forefront during the COVID pandemic, but the points that it raised are transferable outside of pandemic restrictions.

Al-Osaimi and Fawaz (2022) recognise that the right blend of face-to-face instruction and online delivery can improve students' academic achievement but only if the student is engaged in that learning activity.

'Starting anything new is nerve-wracking, and whilst the thought of undertaking some learning online was not worrying in itself, the bigger picture of what that entailed was a cause for worry. Due to the pandemic, we started year 1 online and spent most of that year receiving theoretical content online, distanced from our University campus. What this meant in practical terms was different to a non-pandemic experience or the experience that a student starting year 2 would have if they had already had a year on campus. Students 'arrive' at university with different skills, experiences, and levels of confidence; the student body are a diverse range of students from diverse backgrounds. "Our" cohort had a higher proportion of mature students which also brings a range of challenges which could affect how different students feel about online studying'.

- Jennie Brady, third-year child nursing student, University of Bradford

Technology and the 'art of studying' are both very important aspects. In today's age, would it be considered 'the norm' for all students studying at university to be proficient and computer literate? For all the students at the same level of ability?

Potentially, many students will not have access to appropriate IT or reliable Wi-Fi off campus—this needs to be considered if there is an expectation you will be required to work online (Table 2.3).

TIP

- Be ready and be aware of what is required
- Have your secure login details ready
- Ensure you have contacted relevant IT departments ahead of online sessions for help
- Know how your equipment works and have a practice run
- Identify how you can motivate yourself to succeed

TABLE 2.3 IMPORTANT POINTS TO CONSIDER SUPPORTING YOUR ONLINE LEARNING

Questions to ask yourself	Points to be considered
<ul><li>Do you have a suitable learning environment to enable you to participate?</li><li>Where is your workspace located?</li><li>Are you in a specific study space or in a busy kitchen or living room?</li><li>Do you need to clear all your equipment away at mealtimes?</li></ul>	<ul><li>Wherever possible, create a study space that will be dedicated to you, one where you can leave it all set up for the next session.</li><li>Think about lighting and the position of your desk and yourself to this.</li><li>Think about how you can maximise on natural light.</li><li>You need to make sure the space is the right temperature for you.</li><li>Do you have good access to refreshments</li></ul>
<ul><li>Are you confident with your IT skills?</li><li>Do you see IT as a barrier or as an enabler?</li><li>Can you get the support online to help with setting up for online learning?</li></ul>	<ul><li>If you have a new laptop/desktop, ensure you have figured out how to use it before the classes start.</li><li>Make sure you have the required software uploaded: Microsoft Teams, Office, OneDrive, etc.</li><li>If you feel you would benefit from this, identify IT sessions at university that you can attend.</li><li>Be aware of IT support—do you have an IT drop-in provision on campus? Identify beforehand how to access this.</li><li>Develop your own strategy for remembering usernames and login details—these are your details</li></ul>
<ul><li>How do I maintain motivation if I'm studying alone?</li><li>What social aspects do you need to be mindful of?</li></ul>	<ul><li>Consider setting up peer support groups on social media to reach out to each other and to reduce any potential feelings of isolation.</li><li>Think about how you can keep yourself focused and engaged with the session.</li><li>If you are in a group session, have your camera on and be present.</li><li>Prepare for online study as if you were on campus, get up, get dressed, etc.</li></ul>

TABLE 2.3 IMPORTANT POINTS TO CONSIDER SUPPORTING YOUR ONLINE LEARNING—cont'd

Questions to ask yourself	Points to be considered
• Are there any financial concerns?	• Have adequate access to appropriate equipment at home. Widening participation has introduced more students than ever to a university education (McLellan et al., 2016), but this does not automatically mean all families are financially resourced the same. • Look at any support funding you may be eligible to receive.
• Do you have a confirmed learning disability?	• Ensure your disability assessment is current and includes provision for online study. Seek timely supervision from your disability advisor to help with your online study.

What is the best way to approach online study?

CASE STUDY

Elsie is a first-year learning disabilities nursing student and, during a workshop, is tasked in her group to identify as many different approaches to online study as they can. Elsie has previously struggled with knowing where to start with working together online and is anxious about taking part. The students are encouraged to undertake a group discussion to explore online study in more depth and to provide a summary of the points they discussed. Elsie makes some notes of the points:

• Setting out a specific time to do the work
• Making sure you have a comfortable place to work that is warm and ventilated and has sufficient natural light
• Has taken efforts to avoid any disturbances

Continued

CASE STUDY—cont'd

- Make sure everyone is clear about what is required. What are the learning outcomes for this activity?

Elsie identified that the group discussion identified a lot of the same points that she had thought about. This demonstrated to Elsie that how she was feeling and the worries she had were all real and very valid.

It is important to develop a mindset whereby an online class has the same significance and importance as a class that is delivered face to face. It is not an optional class, and therefore, it is a mandatory component of the programme. This addresses points such as professionalism and presentation of self. The NMC (2023) standards for pre-registration nursing programmes exist to illustrate what is required of you as you progress to registration. These standards of professionalism must be upheld not only in the placement area but within the university context as well. This is about addressing the psychological needs associated with motivation, as discussed by Al-Osaimi and Fawaz (2022). Motivation can slip as courses progress (Rafii et al., 2019), so you need to be able to recognise when your motivation is starting to reduce and how you can successfully manage that. It is important to allow yourself time to prepare for an online class; get up, get dressed, have your notes ready and ensure any pre-reading has been completed. As already discussed, having a designated work area is of huge importance and can contribute to your learning success. However, in situations where you might have to pack away your 'uni stuff' in order to use the table for dinner, make sure your equipment is not moved so far away as to create a problem when you next come to work online.

TIP

- Develop a mindset where you are present
- Be ready for the class
- Check you have the online links and that it works
- Make sure your preparation work is complete
- Present yourself online as you would in the classroom

Is online study enjoyable?

CASE STUDY

Bilal, a first-year mental health nursing student, was talking with some of his peers about their thoughts of online learning; did they enjoy it, or did they think it was a waste of time? Bilal was interested by this because he wasn't really sure how he felt, and he recognised how he struggled to get involved. He always wanted to be there but found it difficult to engage. Some of Bilal's peers explained that they felt the same way and that they should work together to see how they could motivate each other. In their small group, they devised a list of positive and negative points, which they all contributed to. By completing these lists, they could see how positive and productive online learning and teaching can be.

There are many enjoyable aspects of online learning, such as:

- No long commute or battling rush hour traffic
- At break or lunch, you have the opportunity to relax more easily, perhaps undertake some domestic tasks rather than doing it after a long day at university, etc.
- Financially, it saves money to be at home, considering fuel, parking, and a dog walker!
- Lack of interruption
- You are able to concentrate on the lecture undisturbed by the late arrivals or other students talking, etc.

There are some issues with online learning as well:

- The missed opportunity for discussion with peers is a significant disadvantage, this may be debate or listening to other questions within the lecture or in the informal setting of the lunchroom.
- Making friends doesn't happen online as easily, and those relationships are vital for support throughout the whole degree. This is very significant. Peer support is important in so many ways, as described by Cust and Guest (2020). Good peer support can lead to improved leadership, increased self-esteem, improved knowledge, better networking and improved confidence. Cust and

Guest (2020) have also identified how a good peer relationship can have a massive positive impact on student mental health; this needs to be considered in any online classroom and strive to make peer relationships as effective as possible, perhaps in a different way, but with the same or similar outcomes.

TIP

- Make sure those around you know it is demanding work. You are studying at a degree level, even if you are on your sofa—you're not just at home, so make sure they support you!
- Have a bottle and snack with you.
- Get your camera on and join in—it is nerve-wracking, but the sooner you do it, the easier it becomes, and the more you engage, the more you get out of it.
- Take your breaks and lunch away from your computer or screen—get some fresh air, make a cuppa, do what makes you feel good for that break.

Working with others

Peer support within this context is the beginning of your professional working relationships, which will increase and widen in the coming years. To start developing professional relationships now is greatly encouraged so that you can provide support, friendship and care to each other.

Already within this chapter, we have acknowledged the findings of Cust and Guest (2020), who were able to identify a great number of benefits resulting from positive peer relationships. This support is very positively regarded, and you may find that you have these relationships already; you just don't call them peer relationships—are they your 'BFFs'?

Moving forward, it is important to broaden the horizons of working with others, for example, looking at the practice areas where you will undertake your placements. The benefits interprofessional working can bring for your patients, clients, service users, families and other professionals, as well as for your own professional development, are considerable (Grant and Goodman, 2019).

What does 'working with others' mean to you?

As already discussed in this book, building support networks is vital for nursing students to foster personal growth, gain professional guidance and navigate the challenges of nursing studies successfully. You may have the opportunity to work with academics to develop theoretical teaching content based on your and your peers' feedback. Take this chance; if you do, this partnership working will enhance your learning journey and strengthen peer and professional relationships.

CASE STUDY

Ruby and some of her first-year mental health nursing student peers collectively explore the principles around working together. Before starting her nursing degree course, Ruby knew that there were many different types of healthcare professionals but was unsure who they all were and how they all got involved in patient care. They decided to see how many different members of healthcare professionals they could identify, as well as recognising the benefits of learning and growing together.

Throughout your nursing programme, you'll collaborate with various professionals, caring for patients in different ways (Fig 2.2). Teamwork, whether within a group of individuals with similar or different professional backgrounds, is the key to improving patient outcomes (Grant and Goodman, 2019). Benefits from interprofessional working are particularly important, supporting comprehensive and integrated care by breaking down professional silos and promoting a person-centred holistic approach to healthcare delivery (Botten, 2012). It is therefore necessary to start to acquire teamwork knowledge and skills as a student so that they can be developed further in practice and throughout your career. Undertaking placements allows you to learn and grow alongside the interdisciplinary team, helping you understand the benefits of this collaborative approach (Grant and Goodman, 2019). These experiences offer numerous opportunities to enhance professional practices and communication skills and deepen your learning.

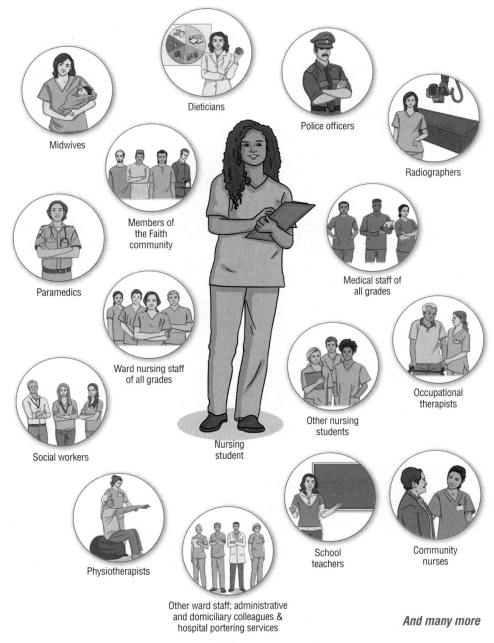

Fig. 2.2   The different professionals.

TIP

- Always remember that everybody is on the team
- Embrace all opportunities to work alongside other peers and other professionals
- Identify what other professionals you are potentially going to meet
- Be aware of the roles and responsibilities of all the different professionals that you meet
- Never be afraid to ask to speak to colleagues about their roles and the contributions they make

What are the advantages and disadvantages of working with others?

CASE STUDY

Sanjay is a first-year adult and mental health nursing student who is preparing for his next summative assignment, titled 'Explore the advantages and disadvantages of working together to enhance patient care'.

Sanjay identified that he needed to understand more about this before he could decide what the advantages and disadvantages were.

Through accessing, reading and reflecting on the relevant literature and his own practice, Sanjay recognised that the following key points would be significant.

- Being part of a team involves both collaborative and independent contributions to ensure success.
- 'Getting people on board' (Geoghegan, 2020, p 21), that is, a shared understanding of the nature of the issue is a fundamental requirement for the success of an activity.
- Working and learning with peers provides the opportunity for psychologically safe spaces to develop personally and professionally whilst feeling supported. Being able to try ideas out, admit you don't understand and learn from others is invaluable (Cust and Guest, 2020).
- Sharing personal experiences as patients, carers and professionals leads to valuable discussions and diverse perspectives, enhancing the overall learning experience and transferable teamwork skills.

Nursing students learn and work together in various settings, gaining valuable experiences along the way. During placements, you will collaborate with peers, identifying challenges in professional relationships, and learn to navigate these situations, fostering personal resilience and effective communication (NMC, 2018a and 2018b). In theoretical modules, your peer relationships may pose challenges due to various factors, such as age, friendship groups, diverse beliefs and opinions. However, both of these situations offer opportunities to develop coping strategies and manage conflicts. Throughout your journey to graduation and beyond, you will share both laughter and tears, forming strong bonds and supporting each other.

 TIP

- Be enquiring
- Be positive and engaging
- Be ready to learn from different professionals
- Be ready to be inspired by different professionals
- Develop your own ability to teach and inspire others to learn and grow together

How can the benefits of working together be maximised to their full potential?

By learning about and using effective strategies and best practices, nursing students can unlock the power of synergy and create a supportive environment that enhances their learning journey and professional growth.

 'As we have progressed through the course the obvious importance of being able to work with others not just at a superficial level but with reflexivity and understanding has become absolutely clear. That understanding was not there at the start of the course, but now in year 3 we are clear about why we are constantly taken out of our comfort zone to challenge ourselves and grow. That ability to engage and interact positively with people is essential. The course nurtures this through team-based

learning, cross allied health sessions, group presentations and assignments to develop that teamwork. To maximise this, students need to be given these opportunities from the very start of the course and to understand the rationale behind it. Students also need to be able to rely on others to share our own desire to achieve and succeed. Students are taught about accountability and the development of this in relation to teamwork is so important, the setting of group rules supports us manage our peer working but is very important for us to have academic support when things aren't working the way they should. It is very hard in a team when you are carrying people and learning how to deal with this as a student is beneficial to us in our professional life'.

- Jennie Brady, third-year child nursing student, University of Bradford

Ellis (2022) and Grant and Goodman (2019) explore many different themes and principles that must be considered when maximising working with others. These include:

Individual roles, responsibility and accountability: Team members need to understand their responsibilities in relation to the task at hand. If someone is not clear about what is being asked, then there is a duty to inform the team leader of this.

Delegation and delegation decisions: Tasks should only be delegated by the person who has responsibility for that task. It is really important that the person who has delegated the task retains responsibility for that task. If this includes a student, then their supervisor will hold that responsibility throughout the duration of that task.

Working with a skills mix: Becoming aware of the different skillsets colleagues have is a big part of working with others. It is important to note that skill sets can change quickly, so it is important to know who is in your team and what their scope of practice is. Students have extremely important contributions to make in terms of taking part in care delivery, but colleagues need to be aware of where students are in their training, as well as their level of competence and requirements for ongoing supervision.

Effective teamworking: This will ensure that patient outcomes are improved and then maintained. Being part of an effective team provides individuals with a sense of belonging and provides many opportunities to work alongside each other towards a shared goal. The NMC (2018a) Future Nurse: Standards of Proficiency for Registered Nurses recognise and emphasise the significance and important of teamwork and each other's responsibilities within those teams. This philosophy nurtures individuals within the team to recognise areas for development and further learning whilst receiving support and help from colleagues around you.

NMC

THE NMC SAYS

8.1. 'Respect the skills and expertise and contributions of your colleagues, referring matter to them when appropriate'.

9. 'Share your skills, knowledge and experience for the benefit of people receiving care and your colleagues'.

11. 'Be accountable for your own decisions to delegate tasks and duties to other people'.

13. 'Recognise and work within the limits of your competence'.

TIP

- Be ready to explore the working relationships that you see in clinical practice as well as in university
- Make the most of every occasion to be part of the team, working together towards a shared goal
- It's OK to talk to team members about working together with different colleagues

CONCLUSION

In this chapter, we have discussed the importance of understanding how you and others learn. We have also discussed how you can optimise your study habits to ensure you are learning as effectively as possible and making the best use of your time. Identifying the strategies that work best for you and then implementing them will help you to achieve your maximum potential in your nursing programme. Nursing programmes can be challenging, so developing these effective study habits can help you to maintain a good study/life balance.

Now you have finished this chapter. Please make notes on what you have learned.

_____

_____

_____

_____

_____

_____

_____

_____

_____

_____

_____

_____

_____

_____

_____

_____

_____

REFERENCES

Allen, S.J. (2007) 'Adult learning theory and leadership development'. *Leadership Review* 7(Spring), pp. 26–37. Available at: https://doi.org/10.1177/10525629211008645

Al-Osaimi, D N. Fawaz, M. (2022) 'Nursing students' perceptions on motivation strategies to enhance academic achievement through blended learning: a qualitative study'. *Helcyon* 8(7), e09818. Available at: doi: 10.1016/j.heliyon.2022.e09818

Botten, E.L. (2012) 'Interprofessional working: the only way forward', *British Journal of Nursing*, 21(9), pp. 549–549. Available at: https://doi.org/10.12968/bjon.2012.21.9.549.

Cirillo, F, (2013) *The Pomodoro Technique*., Berlin: FC Garage.

Cottrell, S. (2019) *The Study Skills Handbook* 5th Edition. London: Red Globe Press.

Cust, F., Guest, K. (2020) 'Peer support for undergraduate children's nursing students'. *Journal of Nursing Education & Practice*, 10(4), pp. 21–25. Available at: https://doi.org/10.5430/jnep.v10n4p21

Ellis, P. (2022) *Leadership management & teamworking in nursing*. Transforming Nursing Practice. Learning Matters. Thousand Oaks: Sage.

Geoghegan, L. (2020) in Swanwick, T Vaux E (ed) *ABC of Quality Improvement in Healthcare*. Hoboken: Wiley Blackwell pp. 21.

Grant, A. and Goodman, B. (2019) (4th ed) *Communication and Interpersonal Skills in Nursing*. Transforming nursing practice. Learning matters. Thousand Oaks: Sage.

Hughes, G. (2020) *Be Well, Learn Well*. London: Red Globe Press.

Judd, T., (2015). 'Task selection, task switching and multitasking during computer-based independent study'. *AJET*, 31(2), pp. 193–207. Available at: https://doi.org/10.14742/ajet.1992

Koriat, A., Bjork, R.A. (2005) 'Illusions of competence in monitoring one's knowledge during study'. *Journal of Experimental Psychology: Learning, Memory and Cognition*, 31(2), pp. 187–194. Available at: https://doi.org/10.1037/0278-7393.31.2.187

Kruger, J. Dunning, D. (1999) 'Unskilled and unaware of it: how difficulties in recognizing one's own incompetence lead to inflated self-assessments'. *Journal of Personality and Social Psychology*, 77(6), pp. 1121–1134. Available at: https://doi.org/10.1037/0022-3514.77.6.1121

McLellan, J. Pettigrew, R. Sperlinger, T. (2016) 'Remaking the elite university: an experiment in widening participation in the UK'. *Power and Education,* Vol 8(1), pp. 54–72. Available at: https://doi.org/10.1177/1757743815624117

Morehead, K., Dunlosky, J., Rawson, K.A. (2019) 'How much mightier is the pen than the keyboard for note-taking? A replication and extension of Mueller and Oppenheimer (2014)', *Educational Psychology Review*, 31(3), pp. 753–780. Available at: https://doi.org/10.1007/s10648-019-09468-2.

Nursing & Midwifery Council (2018a) Future nurse: Standards of proficiency for registered nurses. Available at: https://www.nmc.org.uk/standards/standards-for-nurses/standards-of-proficiency-for registered-nurses/ Accessed 04/08/2023

Nursing & Midwifery Council (2018b) *The Code; Professional standards of practice & behaviour for nurses, midwives and nursing associates*. Available at: https://www.nmc.org.uk/standards/code/. Accessed 04/08/2023

Nursing & Midwifery Council (2023) Standards for pre-registration programmes. Available at: https://www.nmc.org.uk/standards/standards-for-nurses/standards-for-pre-registration-nursing-programmes/ Accessed 04/08/2023

Penn, P. (2020) *The Psychology of Effective Studying*. Abingdon: Routledge.

Rafii, F. Saeedi, M. and Parvizy, S. (2019) 'Academic motivation in nursing students: a hybrid concept analysis'. *Journal of Nursing & Midwifery,* 24(5), pp. 315–322. Available at: DOI: 10.4103/ijnmr.IJNMR_177_18

Rutherford-Hemming, T. (2012) 'Simulation methodology in nursing education and adult learning theory'. *Adult Learning,* 23(3), pp. 129–137. Available at: https://doi.org/10.1177/1045159512452848

Rogers, T. Milkman, K. and Norton, M. (2015) 'Beyond good intentions: prompting people to make plans improves follow-through on important tasks', *Behavioural Science & Policy*, 1(2), pp. 33–41. Available at: https://doi.org/10.1353/bsp.2015.0011.

Wu, J.-Y. and Xie, C. (2018) 'Using time pressure and note-taking to prevent digital distraction behaviour and enhance online search performance: perspectives from the load theory of attention and cognitive control', *Computers in Human Behaviour*, 88, pp. 244–254. Available at: https://doi.org/10.1016/j.chb.2018.07.008.

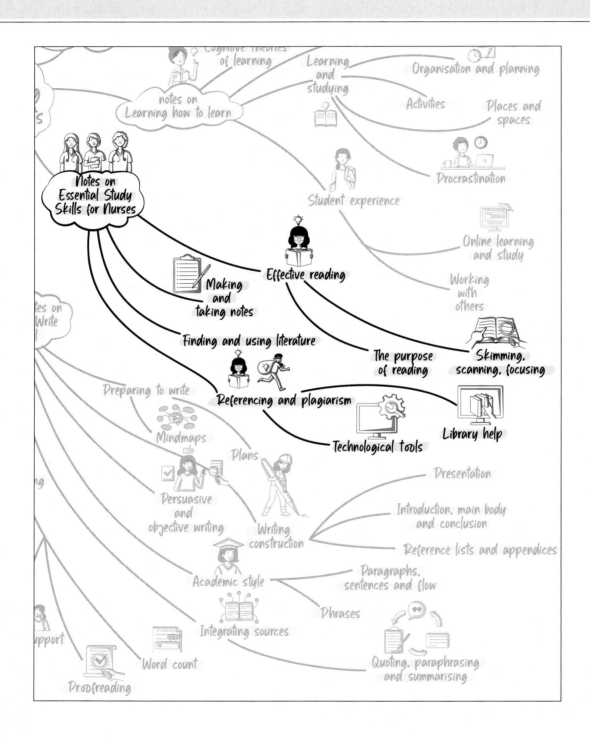

NOTES ON ESSENTIAL STUDY SKILLS FOR NURSES

Anita Z Goldschmied ■ Dean-David Holyoake

INTRODUCTION

Study skills are the building blocks of your nursing practice. This chapter introduces four essential study skills and their relationships as shown in Fig 3.1. (1) how to read effectively, (2) how to take and make notes, (3) how to find and use literature and (4) how to reference and avoid plagiarism. If you master these tools, studying not only becomes more creative but also satisfying and representative of other transferable skills and ideals in your nursing career (NMC, 2018a).

You are here, just about to begin or have just begun your nursing degree. It means you already have a wealth of skills and expertise in studying and a good knowledge of what works for you. We aim to give you some ideas to help you build on your strengths and encourage you to experiment, get curious and improve. Undeniably, some activities, such as referencing, must meet academic expectations, and we will highlight these skills. Yet others are open to adaptation and shaped by your learning style. All four study skills have the same overarching aim: to help you find, engage and evaluate a wide range of information (see Buzan, 2011, for more helpful ideas about brainstorming and mind mapping).

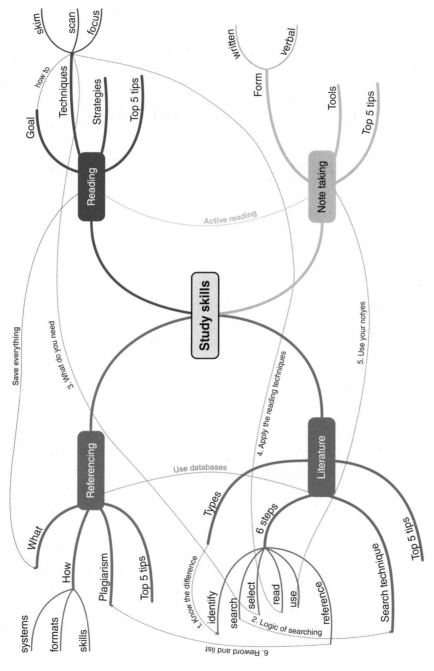

Fig. 3.1   A concept map of the study skills and their relationships.

HOW TO BECOME AN EFFECTIVE READER

Why do I need to improve my reading skills?

You have been reading since infancy, so you might wonder why you need to learn again. Well, you are now reading for a nursing degree, and being a university student demands that you read a lot. In addition, your reading is at another level. As you move from level 4 to level 6 and beyond (see Chapter 6), you are working towards a professional qualification and registration, requiring a growing sense of academic independence, the ability to make connections and a commitment to lifelong learning. Reading, then, is a skill underpinning your academic study and nursing practice.

The good news is that reading skills can continuously be improved in at least two ways. First, it can be divided into expanding language skills (grammar, fluency, vocabulary) and mental skills (attention, focus, reasoning). Second, you can become a more effective reader by engaging with the tools discussed in the following sections (Buzan, 2006). We start from the assumption that you have a good foundation in these skills but are curious to keep testing and challenging yourself.

SOCIAL MEDIA
@WeNurses

'It is great to be curious, it is a fantastic nurse skill too! #Stayandthrive'

The goal of your reading

What are some things you have read and will do during your nursing career? You probably regularly read emails, magazines and social media posts, but there is no doubt that the range of academic materials you will start engaging with will expand. Some publications are written in everyday English, while others use more technically complex and scientific language that you will need to navigate. One way or another, reading forms a massive part of what we nurses do, so make yours amazing and more effective.

Effective reading starts with knowing what you want to read. You need a clear goal, and Table 3.1 is one way of thinking about this. In academic

TABLE 3.1   THE GOAL OF READING

Goal	Theory	Technique	Practice	Example
Mandatory suggested	Mandatory reading is essential and thus must be read. Suggested texts widen your knowledge.	Find and scan the reading lists; then use focused reading for detail.	In module and course handbooks, virtual learning environment, assignment briefs, online library.	Find the mandatory and suggested reading list for your nursing modules.
'How to'	The text explains the steps to achieve a specific aim. It instructs what to do, in what order and where to get more support.	These texts require focused reading. Misunderstanding and missing details can have consequences.	Assignment brief, BNF, aseptic procedure, drug leaflet, how to search literature or submit your assignment.	You have to submit an essay. You need to understand the expectations, learning outcomes and processes.
Overview and explore	The aim is to explore a topic and develop a general awareness. It includes key dates, definitions, activities, people.	Keep the broad topic in mind as you skim through various sources. Do not fixate on specific aspects.	Flipping through the pages of diverse materials such as books, articles, websites, course documents, etc.	You might have a broad title and notes from the lectures. You need to explore the key areas and central issues.

Understand and learn	The aim is to understand, learn and memorise specific skills, procedures, theories and concepts.	Focused reading helps learn the key points, compare views, select definitions and comprehend theories.	You need to use various sources and voices. You identify relevant sections and points and read them carefully.	You narrowed your interest. You need to understand the key theories, data and procedures.
Evidence and detail	Nurses must evidence their actions. The skill is to decide which literature to use and when and how to reference them.	With a specific question in mind, scan the text to decide whether it is relevant, and then understand, learn and apply it.	Evidence comes in many forms: research articles about outcomes, legislation about rights, guides about procedures.	When you explain or apply a theory in your assignment, you need to evidence the sources of your argument.
Apply and connect	Case studies and reflective pieces demonstrate how theory works in practice and what can be done.	You need to use all techniques to show how knowledge and theories apply in a case and context.	Everything nurses do in your essays, presentations, exams, practice documents, care assessments.	Nurses must show how our actions and decisions are evidenced, justified and applied.
Enjoy and inspire	Generally, not academic reading that aims to inspire, motivate or entertain.	Be creative, mix the techniques and build on your strengths. Do more of what you do well.	Quotes, life stories, fiction, podcasts, videos, drawing and even academic materials.	When you need inspiration, browse the web, watch YouTube or read tweets.

BNF, British National Formulary.

reading, we rarely read a book or an article from the beginning to end, word by word. Therefore, having a clear goal (such as understanding an assignment brief) makes reading more productive and even enjoyable. The goal of reading helps you decide what source you need, where you will find the material and what technique is the most useful. As introduced in Chapter 2, your attitude towards the text does half of the job because a curious mindset in motion is one capable of exploring, selecting and storing information.

NMC

THE NMC SAYS

'The confidence and ability to think critically, apply knowledge and skills, and provide expert, evidence-based, direct nursing care therefore lies at the centre of all registered nursing practice'.

SOCIAL MEDIA
@WeNurses

'We love this quote from @readingagency which sums up the power and importance of reading as something to help us practise #selfcareforlife #selfcareweek @selfcareforum

In a world where inequality is widening, where family and community networks are fragmenting and poor health and well-being is reaching epidemic proportions, we need the power of reading more than ever as a tool for change'.

Three fundamental reading techniques

We have categorised the goal of reading into seven types (Table 3.1). These can help you consider your reading in terms of 'actively noticing' and employing different reading techniques. Table 3.2 goes further to explain skimming, scanning and focusing. Mix and match

TABLE 3.2 THREE TYPES OF READING TECHNIQUES

Technique	Aim	Skills	Application
Skimming	To have a general and broad awareness. To decide if you need more detail. To find further relevant material.	Have a broad topic in mind. Flip through the pages to note headings, highlights, things that stand out like tables, lists and keywords. Read the introduction, summaries and conclusion.	**Survey, screen, save** different sources such as books, articles, websites, guides and legislation to explore the broad topic.
Scanning	To find specific information. To decide if you need to learn it. To find evidence, key points and themes.	Have specific keywords or questions in mind. Do not read all paragraphs word by word, but stop at key points. Notice specific expressions, clusters of words, themes.	**Find, select, highlight** key points, expressions, sections, themes, people, data, theories about a more specific aspect of your topic.
Focusing	To understand the text, the concepts, the arguments. To memorise key information. To evidence the work and detail.	Read more carefully, usually word by word. There will be sentences and sections you need to read more than once. Reflect on what you read, jot down queries and ideas, ask questions.	**Read, question, reflect** to have a detailed and evidenced understanding of your topic's theories, definitions, examples and details.

these techniques to help break down reading into smaller pieces. It makes the task of finding and reading literature more accessible and effective.

Skimming is surveying many materials. In the same way you flip through the pages of a magazine, do the same with academic articles, textbooks and research abstracts. Your initial skimming should be an exciting curiosity into the broad topic and not restricted to what you think you already know. The important point to remember as you progress is 'everything read is useful' (even if only to disregard later). Skimming, by its very nature, means collecting, collating and being prepared to return to scan in more detail.

Scanning is narrowing down your interest, for example, to a specific theory or intervention. You can start a more careful and considered scanning of the saved materials to find relevant parts that explain the model, its application and notable people. You also return to skimming as you need to locate more specific materials. In short, you are scanning as a means to select literature for focused reading.

Focusing is reading specific sections or paragraphs you have selected as being essential and is the slowest technique. Whilst this type of reading is laborious, it allows you to fully comprehend the identified parts of the text. Persist. Many clinical guides will require such intricate reading, so it is essential that you become confident and prepared to persist if you do not understand something.

Reading difficult materials

You will encounter both academic and practice materials that will be complicated and unfamiliar. They may have an unusual format and style and often use complex, technical or scientific language. You may be tempted to fall back on your comfort zones: websites and summaries that are easier to understand. This is a natural response, and sometimes reading these materials can give you a general understanding and boost your confidence. However, it is essential that every nurse can navigate diverse literature such as academic books, journal articles, research papers, policies and guides. So, give yourself time to go through difficult texts (Paul and Elder, 2019). From day 1, make sure you have access to an English dictionary, and expect that many nursing texts contain numbers and complex formulas (if necessary, skim through statistics), requiring more time to comprehend. Sometimes reading a text out loud helps comprehension.

The more you employ a system of reading, the sooner you will start making it work for yourself.

From passive to active reading

For some, reading can be a tedious and boring exercise and a perfect excuse to catch yourself planning dinner. So, what are the steps you can take to make your reading more of an active performance? See Fig. 3.2.

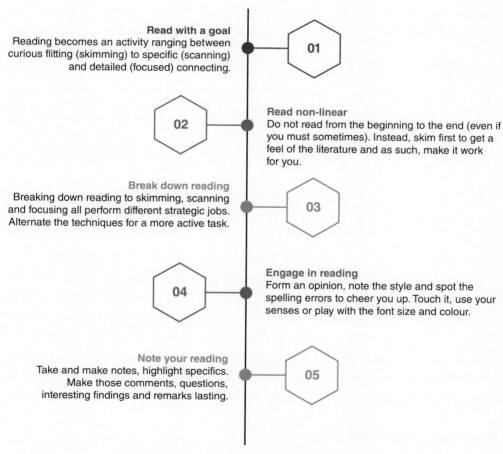

FROM PASSIVE TO ACTIVE READING

Read with a goal
Reading becomes an activity ranging between curious flitting (skimming) to specific (scanning) and detailed (focused) connecting.

01

02

Read non-linear
Do not read from the beginning to the end (even if you must sometimes). Instead, skim first to get a feel of the literature and as such, make it work for you.

Break down reading
Breaking down reading to skimming, scanning and focusing all perform different strategic jobs. Alternate the techniques for a more active task.

03

04

Engage in reading
Form an opinion, note the style and spot the spelling errors to cheer you up. Touch it, use your senses or play with the font size and colour.

Note your reading
Take and make notes, highlight specifics. Make those comments, questions, interesting findings and remarks lasting.

05

Fig. 3.2 Five steps to move from passive to active reading.

TIP

Top 5 tips for effective reading

- Always read with a clear goal and aim.
- Learn, mix and match the reading techniques.
- Stay creative and break down the reading into smaller tasks.
- Apply the various strategies of active reading.
- Make an English-English dictionary your best friend.

Reflect on your reading experiences, skills and ideals. How can you become more confident in reading difficult and complex academic literature?

_____

_____

_____

_____

THE ART OF MAKING AND TAKING NOTES

If effective reading is one of the most essential skills that will make your nursing journey more successful, note-taking comes a close second. We have already hinted at how important notes are in making reading an interactive activity rather than a passive exercise. Note-taking is the act of noticing, recording and summarising key points and information from written or verbal literature. Notes serve more than one purpose. They can help you outline, summarise, analyse, compare and contrast, evidence, pattern and memorise. See Fig. 3.3.

Note-taking strategies and skills

The note-taking strategies and skills introduced in this section, together with the reading skills, will make your studying, writing and observing more effective in academia and practice. To start, note-taking strategies

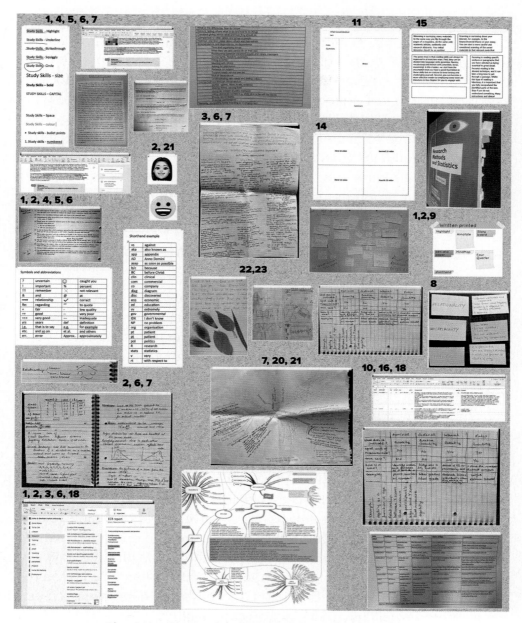

Fig. 3.3 Note-taking examples from our works.

can be grouped together based on the type of material: physical and printed materials, virtual and electronic and verbal and mixed audio materials. There are other ways of thinking about notes, such as their format (handwritten, typed, artistic, voice recorded) and their logic (linear, systematic, mapping).

Some tools are better for certain purposes than others, but do not limit how you take notes. During a presentation or on placement, you need quick and efficient strategies. You rarely have the time to spread 50 coloured pencils on the table. Whilst at home, when preparing for your assignment, you will need to work yourself through dozens of books, articles and complex texts. These are the moments when you have freedom and time to experiment and use your strengths and preferred learning styles (Marks-Beale, 2002). We often think we will remember things until we realise days later that our initial ideas resemble alien communication. Good note-taking ensures that our notes make sense when we need them most. See Table 3.3.

Note-taking from printed and physical materials

These materials are physical, and examples include printed books, articles, instructions, guides such as the British National Formulary, care plans, assessment forms, photos and life stories written by people with lived experience. You might find that printing electronic materials helps your reading and comprehension. Most of us find that these materials are the easiest to access. The only problem is if you lose them (please see chapter 10), spill your coffee on them or leave them on the sofa and your new family member, Aston, the puppy, eats them.

Note-taking from virtual and electronic materials

Your university library allows you access to electronic materials; whilst on placement, you will write care plans and read notes electronically. Digital materials and note-taking have a weightless advantage that makes them accessible even if they do require some digital skills and sometimes specialist equipment (see Chapter 7 on digital literacy). You will probably need to learn more than one software and their features. Most of the tools you use in printed and physical materials, such as a highlighter pen, will have an electronic equivalent.

Note-taking from verbal and mixed audio materials

Most of your face-to-face lectures, seminars and online teaching will fall into this category. You will also have regular handovers and meetings in practice with minimal or no written materials available. Podcasts, videos

TABLE 3.3 TRADITIONAL NOTE-TAKING APPROACHES

Method	TYPE OF MATERIAL			NOTE-TAKING		
	Printed	Virtual	Verbal	Difficulty	Logic	Form
Colours, sizes, space, shape Combine them and develop a system to help organise, highlight and manage your notes.	✓	✓	✓	★ EASY	L	D,H,P
Symbols, shorthand, abbreviations Download existing systems and make them yours. Use the common signs such as: !, ?, +, i.e.,	✓	✓	✓	★★ MEDIUM	L	D,H,P
Outline, sentence and bullet point Use headings and other pointers. Limit the number of topics. Leave space for flexibility.	✓	✓	✓	★ EASY	L	D,H
Highlight (underline, strike out) Focus on key points. Things you do not understand. Use colours systematically.	✓	✓		★ EASY	L	D,H
Annotations Add words, sentences, questions. Build a system and use symbols. Jot down ideas so you do not lose momentum.	✓	✓		★★ MEDIUM	L	D,H

Continued

TABLE 3.3 TRADITIONAL NOTE-TAKING APPROACHES—cont'd

| Method | TYPE OF MATERIAL | | | NOTE-TAKING | | |
	Printed	Virtual	Verbal	Difficulty	Logic	Form
Notepads and notebooks Be inspired by funky, colourful, sparkling decorations in exciting shapes and sizes. Use it creatively.	✓	✓	✓	★ EASY	L,S,M	D,H,P
Pen and paper Make sure you number the pages. You can attach them more flexibly than notebooks. Use various sizes and colours.	✓	✓	✓	★ EASY	L,S,M	H
Cards You can freely group, move and rearrange them. Use colours, sizes and shapes to have more fun and usefulness. Cards have two sides!	✓	✓	✓	★ EASY	S,M	D,H,P
Post-it Like cards but with one side only. You can stick them onto a surface or use them as a page marker.	✓	✓		★ EASY	S,M	D,H,P

Logic: *L*, Linear; *M*, mapping; *S*, systematic. Form: *D*, Digital version is possible; *H*, possible to create on paper/notebook; *P*, specific program is available.

and animation are more and more popular. Recordings of interviews, performances, conference presentations and even the radio might be a key source. These materials often give you limited or no opportunity at all to read the actual text or listen to it again (you use fewer senses). These sources can be the most challenging when it comes to note-taking, so be prepared and have a tool or two ready to use. See Table 3.4.

Linear, systematic and mapping approaches

Linear notes are written in a sequence, line after line, page after page, often in a hierarchy. They can have headings, subheadings and other pointers, but they generally move along in succession. They are the easiest way to record notes but the most difficult to organise into themes and relationships. Systematic notes provide you with a template to make your notes more organised and considered. They reveal more relationships, patterns and creative options. Mapping approaches are the most flexible and allow you to create notes using a range of techniques (i.e., drawings, mind maps) and styles (i.e., symbols). These notes require some practice. The mapping style is the best for analysing how things relate and creating themes. See Table 3.5.

SOCIAL MEDIA
@wenurses

'@AndreaJohns20 tweets as your notes! Look on it as note taking, then easy to tweet and listen...... #PHPconf2014'

TIP

Top 5 tips for effective note-taking

1. Highlight and summarise rather than copy and paste.
2. Learn various techniques and combine them.
3. Do not worry about grammar, spelling or style.
4. Use colours, shapes and creative elements.
5. Employ templates and practice the tools.

TABLE 3.4 STRUCTURED NOTE-TAKING

Method	TYPE OF MATERIAL			NOTE-TAKING		
	Printed	Virtual	Verbal	Difficulty	Logic	Form
Templates Preformatted sheets. Divide the sheet into parts. Adaptable to suit needs.	✓	✓	✓	★★ MEDIUM	S	D,H,P
Cornell Use three parts (notes, cues, summary). Organises notes into sections.	✓	✓	✓	★ EASY	S	D,H
Q notes Use three parts (questions, answers, reflection). Turn titles into questions. Help focusing and reflecting on key points and your learning.	✓	✓	✓	★★ MEDIUM	S	D,H
QEC method Use three parts (questions, evidence, conclusion). Useful for specific topics. Help critical exploration to arrive at a conclusion.	✓	✓	✓	★★ MEDIUM	L	D,H
Four quarter Use four parts of 15 minutes. Help break down the material. Help focusing on key points.	✓	✓	✓	★ EASY	S	D,H

Method	Difficulty	Logic	Form
Boxing — Separate topics into boxes. Use as many boxes as you wish. Combine it with other tools.	★ EASY	S	D,H
Tables, spreadsheets, charting — Use columns and rows. Use colours, headings, different font types and sizes. Need an idea of the broad design in advance.	★★★ HARD	S	D,H,P
Process maps and flows — Organised and linear maps. Use different shapes, colours. Use arrows and directions.	★★★ HARD	M	D,H,P
Matrix — A special type of table. Focuses on relationships, similarities and differences. Best for specialised subjects.	★★★ HARD	S	D,H
Pyramids — Good for hierarchy. Use various sizes and colours.	★★ MEDIUM	S	D,H
Mind maps — Have a central idea. It requires learning some skills. Use colours, shapes, pictures and anything else.	★★★ HARD	M	D,H,P
Concept maps — Often used interchangeably with mind maps. More structured, less colourful and less artistic.	★★★ HARD	M	D,H,P

Logic: *L*, Linear; *M*, mapping; *S*, systematic. Form: *D*, Digital version is possible; *H*, possible to create on paper/notebook; *P*, specific program is available.

TABLE 3.5 CREATIVE NOTE-TAKING

Method	Type of Material			Note-taking		
	Printed	Virtual	Verbal	Difficulty	Logic	Form
Storyboard Draw, use photos and cartoons. Tell the key points visually. Use templates, boxes and defined spaces to help focus.	✓	✓		★★ MEDIUM	S,M	D,H,P
Drawing and sketching Use stick and simple figures. Help you learn in your way. Practice and develop your style.	✓	✓	✓	★★ MEDIUM	M	D,H,P
Emoji Use to tell stories, highlight key points or other ways to personalise notes.	✓	✓		★★ MEDIUM	L	D,H,P
Voice and video recording Get your phone and press the voice or video recorder to tell your notes, questions, ideas.	✓	✓	✓	★ EASY	L	D,H,P
Photographs Cut out pictures from magazines, add stickers, insert photos to make your note live.	✓	✓		★ EASY	L	D,H,P

Screenshots

Record the page for further work.

Make sure you name and organise them.

| | ★ EASY | L | D,P |

Create and innovate

What about having an avatar?

Do you like singing?

Are you playing an instrument?

Have you tried to write a poem about a theory?

How about reinventing your fridge magnets?

Creating acronyms?

Tweeting, posting and blogging?

Use your self, skills, hobbies and interests whenever you can.

Adapt the tools so they work for you.

| | ★★ MEDIUM | L,S,M | D,H,P |

Logic: *L*, Linear; *M*, mapping; *S*, systematic. Form: *D*, Digital version is possible; *H*, possible to create on paper/notebook; *P*, specific program is available.

Reflect on your note-taking skills. What are the two to three note-taking approaches you are confident with? Can you identify two to three new note-taking techniques that enhance your study skills?

_____

_____

_____

_____

GAINING CONFIDENCE

So far, you have learnt two interlinked skills, active reading and note-taking. Reading and note-taking are such an integrated system that you will find many combined techniques (SQ4R, PQ3R, SQ3R). Mastering these skills means you can explore, analyse, summarise and assemble various materials. But what are the materials we are talking about? The following two skills will cover literature and referencing. Literature is the academic term for the various materials you will read. When you take notes from the literature and use them, you must tell your reader what you accessed. Where do your notes come from? Where do your knowledge and evidence come from? We have a word and a system for this activity. It is called referencing. The rest of the chapter introduces these two essential interlinked nursing skills.

FINDING AND USING LITERATURE

You might wonder why academics and practitioners are so obsessed with literature and referencing. Literature has at least two definitions. First, the broader term refers to any materials you read and use in your studies and practice. Table 3.6 gives you a summary of the different types of literature. Second, and in a narrower sense, literature is often divided into academic literature, which is evidence-based materials using established, formal commercial channels for distribution, and grey literature, which includes everything else usually requiring less controlled, informal publication processes (Schöpfel & Farace, 2015; Rexroth, 2023).

TABLE 3.6 THE VARIOUS TYPES OF LITERATURE

Type	Source	Key Characteristics	Finding	Reading	Priority
Textbook (A)	UL,B,W	Practical books written to students about a topic or profession.	LOW	LOW	HIGH
Academic books (A)	UL,B	Written by experts using more complex language to advance a field.	MEDIUM	MEDIUM	MEDIUM
Generic books (G)	B,W	Used less in academia and practice, written by organisations or individuals.	LOW	LOW	LOW
Research article (A)	UL	Essential to find evidence, best practice examples and other studies.	HIGH	HIGH	HIGH
Academic papers (A)	UL,W	Various publications: reviews, service users' voice, case studies, opinions.	MEDIUM	HIGH	HIGH
Professional papers (G)	UL,W	Primarily written by practice professionals and industry.	MEDIUM	MEDIUM	MEDIUM
Academic journals (A)	UL	Collect research studies, academic papers and other communications.	LOW	HIGH	HIGH
Professional journals (G)	UL,W	Published by originations on contemporary trends and topics.	MEDIUM	MEDIUM	MEDIUM
Conference papers (G)	UL,W	Specific topics prepared for and presented at a conference.	MEDIUM	MEDIUM	LOW
Lecture slides (G)	UL,VLE,W	Prepared by academics to students. Some presentations are shared online.	LOW	LOW	HIGH

Continued

TABLE 3.6 THE VARIOUS TYPES OF LITERATURE—cont'd

Type	Source	Key Characteristics	Finding	Reading	Priority
Legislation (G)	W	Laws that apply to a specific country. Easy-read versions are published.	★ LOW	★★★ HIGH	★★★ HIGH
National policies (G)	W	Essential guides that apply to a large group of people or organisations.	★ LOW	★★ MEDIUM	★★★ HIGH
Local policies (G)	W	Essential guides specific to an environment, organisation or field.	★ LOW	★★ MEDIUM	★★ MEDIUM
Clinical guides (G)	W	Focus on specific issues, conditions, skills or procedures.	★★ MEDIUM	★★ MEDIUM	★★ MEDIUM
Generic guides (G)	W	These come in many forms and shapes, focusing on generic topics.	★ LOW	★ LOW	★ LOW
Regulations (G)	W	Specific organisations who were given rights to write and publish regulations.	★ LOW	★ LOW	★★★ HIGH
Organisations (G)	W	Organisations research, write guides and amplify the members' voices.	★ LOW	★ LOW	★★ MEDIUM
Thesis, essays (G)	UL,W	Most works submitted by students are stored by universities.	★★ MEDIUM	★ LOW	★ LOW
Video (G)	W	Visual (images and/or audio) academic and nonacademic materials.	★★ MEDIUM	★ LOW	★★ MEDIUM
Podcasts (G)	W	Audio-only academic and nonacademic recordings.	★★ MEDIUM	★★ MEDIUM	★★ MEDIUM

Source	Location			Rating
Presentations (G)	UL,VLE,W	Specifically created for an audience to introduce a topic using slides.	★★ MEDIUM	★ LOW	★★ MEDIUM
Opinions (G)	UL,W	Anyone can express one's view on a topic, question or issue.	★ LOW	★ LOW	★ LOW
Blogs (G)	W	Personal pieces that can be written by anyone, including academics.	★★ MEDIUM	★ LOW	★ LOW
Social media (G)	W	Public domain to network, share information and form groups.	★ LOW	★ LOW	★ LOW
News (G)	B,W	Specific papers and websites that cover current affairs written by journalists.	★ LOW	★ LOW	★ LOW
Governmental sources (G)	W	Official publications like policies, data and guides for a country/countries.	★ LOW	★★ MEDIUM	★★ MEDIUM
Charities (G)	W	Not-for-profit organisations with a well-defined aim and target population.	★ LOW	★ LOW	★★ MEDIUM
Think tanks (G)	W	Independent organisations that publish research, guide and other literature.	★ LOW	★ LOW	★★ MEDIUM

A, Academic literature; B, (book)shop; G, grey literature; UL, university library; VLE, virtual learning environment; W, web.

A word on the terminologies used in nursing

As you progress in your nursing career, you will notice differing perspectives, theories and ways of categorising. You will see those various professions reference and define primary and secondary sources, academic and grey literature differently. If you are confused at times, it is probably not you. Psychologists, sociologists, historians and medics use different terminologies, so do not be put off when browsing the web or reading articles. Even within nursing, the various fields (adult, children, mental health and learning disabilities) have slightly different approaches, so be prepared (Goldschmied et al., 2021).

CASE STUDY

Whilst on a community placement, Peter, a Sheffield Hallam University learning disability nursing and social work student, and his practice supervisor visit Rohan, who lives in supported living with two young men. Rohan has a mild learning disability and cerebral palsy and communicates his needs using words, sounds and gestures. Rohan's hip has deteriorated, and he is in constant pain. Rohan was referred to a surgeon who declined the surgery. The doctor felt that hip replacement would not enhance Rohan's quality of life. Rohan expressed that he would like surgery. A multidisciplinary meeting is scheduled. Peter is asked to prepare a case for Rohan.

Peter visits Rohan and explores his views. Peter talks to the staff and reads the care plan. Peter needs information about Rohan's condition, the treatment options and the possible outcomes. Peter searches the internet, goes to the NICE website (www.nice.org.uk) and downloads guides on hip replacement (NICE 2020). Peter visits the university library for books on learning disability to explore Rohan's rights and quality of life. Peter revisits the Mental Capacity Act (2005) (www.legislation.gov.uk) to act in the best interest of Rohan. Peter is still unsure how safe and beneficial this procedure is, so he searches online databases (CINAHL, MEDLINE). He saves research articles about hip replacement, pain management and people with a learning disability.

CASE STUDY—cont'd

Peter skims and scans through books, websites, guides, academic studies and research papers. He focuses his reading on essential information about the pros and cons of hip surgery and quality of life matters. Peter takes notes, highlights key points and records his thoughts in his digital notebook as he prepares a draft case for the meeting. At the multidisciplinary meeting, the health and care professionals discuss Rohan's case. Peter, with the support of his supervisor, presents his argument in favour of hip surgery, which is now supported by a variety of literature and evidence. The 1-hour-long meeting ends with all professionals (adult nurse, learning disability nurse, student nurse, care manager, advocate, physiotherapist, surgeon, anaesthesiologist) supporting Rohan's surgery.

This case study illustrates that academic and professional literature is fundamental to your nursing journey. Fig. 3.4 summarises four essential skills in working with literature. We have covered two activities already ([1] goal and [3] use). The remaining chapter explores how to search for literature ([2] search) and reference ([4] acknowledge).

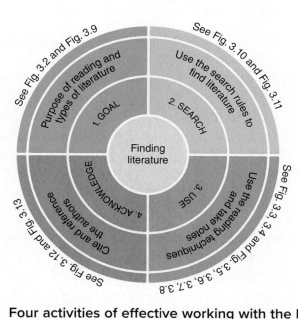

Fig. 3.4   Four activities of effective working with the literature.

NMC

THE NMC SAYS

1.10 'Demonstrate resilience and emotional intelligence and be capable of explaining the rationale that influences their judgments and decisions in routine, complex and challenging situations'.

Searching and finding relevant literature

Whether you use the web or the university library, search engines follow a specific logic. We do not have the room to explain all the nuances of searching here, but there are a few skills we can introduce. The more you understand how algorithms work, the more efficient your searches become. Like reading, this is a skill you will be using forever, so knowing how to search makes your time efficient, your work reliable and your results specific. You need to familiarise yourself with things like keywords, Boolean operators and filters. These rules form the basis of a literature search.

Your primary place to search for academic sources is your university's online library. It gives you access to academic journals, papers and textbooks organised into databases that are not freely available on the web. Academic databases are based on specific professions or topics. CINAHL Complete gives access to nursing-related outputs.

Your secondary source will be the internet to find organisations, legislation and other sources. Google Scholar collects professional and academic output. Open-access academic articles have become more popular, and you can access them online without your university's subscription. However, you will not succeed if most of your sources and literature come from the web because they are limited in scope. Access to most academic outputs is still restricted to paid journals and databases.

CASE STUDY

So how did Peter search relevant academic literature to prepare Rohan's case for the multidisciplinary meeting? He accessed Sheffield Hallam University's online library and searched databases like CINAHL to find a variety of academic outputs.

CASE STUDY—cont'd

Peter started by formulating the broad topic/title/question: what are the benefits and risks of hip replacement for adults with a learning disability?

Then he used specific rules to turn his question into searchable information. We organised the fundamental search rules for you in Fig. 3.5, giving one example from the case study and a brief definition. Peter created many tables combining various rules to explore alternatives and find the best available evidence.

SYNONYMS, ANTONYIMS, AND ACRONYMS
Similar and opposite in meaning to your keywords and abbreviations: intellectual disability is a synonym to learning disability, child is an antonym to adults, LD is an acronym for learning disability.

KEYWORDS
Words created from the topic/title/question and used in the search engine: hip replacement, learning disability, adults, benefits, risks.

SYMBOLS
Instruct the search engine to do something.
* replace characters (Disabilit* for both disability and disabilities)
? spelling variations (person-cent?red for both person-centred or person-centered)
""exact phrase ("hip replacement")

BROADENING AND NARROWING
Alternative words that help extend or narrow down your results. Disability is broader than learning disability, whilst cerebral palsy is narrower.

FILTERS
Different options by the database to narrow down the results.
Date range (2010–2023)
Type (book, article)
Available (online, peer-reviewed)

BOOLEAN OPERATORS
Tell the search engine the relationship between words.
AND – search for both words
OR – search for any of the words
NOT – exclude the word
("Hip replacement") AND ("learning disabilit* OR LD OR "intellectual disability") AND (adult NOT child*).

Fig. 3.5   Essential rules for your literature search.

Skills in literature searching

Finding relevant literature can be daunting and time-consuming. Break it into subtasks and develop a strategy like the one in the case study. Make notes of what you have done by recording your steps and results. When the search engine returns the hits, read the title and decide whether it is relevant. If it seems to be useful, read the abstract or summary. If it still looks suitable, save the document and use the reading skills we discussed at the beginning of this chapter. As you are getting the results, amend your strategy using the rules. Repeat this process using different databases and the web if appropriate until you are satisfied. Whilst using CINAHL Complete, the nursing database, is good practice, you should not rely on this one database only. It is likely that other disciplines, such as allied health professionals, psychology, medics and social scientists, researched and explored hip replacement. You will also notice that when you download a paper or book, they often have weird names or only numbers. Give them a meaningful name, such as hip replacement 1. Create folders, bookmarks and a system for your literature or use existing ones.

SOCIAL MEDIA
@ProfJuneG

'Q1. Study. Whether formal or informal – studying your subject is the only way to develop your knowledge #WeNurses'

TIP

Top 5 tips for effective working with literature

1. Learn how to use the university's online library to find academic literature.
2. Learn the types of literature and when to use them.
3. Learn the logic of search engines to save time and be accurate.
4. Access your university library's support and guides.
5. Learn to enjoy the adventure of searching and finding literature.

REFERENCING AND PLAGIARISM IN ACADEMIA AND PRACTICE

So, what is referencing and plagiarism, and why are we so preoccupied with it? Referencing is the activity of showing the literature you accessed, read and used. Plagiarism is the failure to name the authors and the sources or acknowledge them accurately. There is a difference between cheating when you use other people's works as if they were yours and inaccurate referencing, but both can have similar serious consequences (APA, 2022).

NMC

THE NMC SAYS

20.1 'Keep to and uphold the standards and values set out in the Code'.

20.4 'Keep to the laws of the country in which you are practicing'.

20.8 'Act as a role model of professional behaviour for students and newly qualified nurses, midwives and nursing associates to aspire to'.

The significance of referencing

Right now, we are sitting in front of a computer, thinking about what to write, typing this chapter and creating figures to help you master some study skills. We could be watching the TV or having a drink by the pool somewhere in Spain. We write this chapter for many reasons, mainly because we are passionate about our professions and love our students. We also spent many years and hours studying these skills. If you read, learn or evidence a point, it is not a big request to acknowledge the people and organisations who did the work. But there is another important reason. Sources and sources, literature and literature are not the same. When you write about a theory in your assignment, when you suggest an intervention in practice or when you learn a clinical skill, we need to know where your knowledge comes from. Whilst 100% safe and reliable literature does not exist, we need to be able to trust your information. Hence, we have spent so much time already talking about reading, sources and types of literature.

There is nothing wrong with reading Wikipedia to have an idea about a topic. We all do. However, as a nursing student, you will be in serious trouble if you treat a patient based on those articles without further scrutiny. In your personal life, you have the right to make many decisions, even if they are unwise. We have legislation for this, the Mental Capacity Act (2005). As a professional, you do not have the same freedom. You are responsible for other people's health. You must practice as safely as possible, within reasonable limits, as in real life, you will never be entirely sure. We have highlighted that if you do not use academic literature in your work and practice, you most likely will end up with poor results and even fail. And the reason for this is just that simple: you need to show that you understand the different types of literature, who produces them and what they can do and cannot do—in short, when and how they can be used (NMC, 2018b).

SOCIAL MEDIA
@WeNurses

'Both. For example, we had to do a level 5 30 credit module on PCC and approaches. Lots of material needed to be read and referencing. I have been able to use this to make some solid PBS with my lads. But also, philosophically and encouraging and leading others to do the same'.

Once you understand the significance of referencing, there are two skills left: (1) what to reference, and (2) how to reference to avoid plagiarism. Put this another way. Do you remember how many times we said be creative, use your skills and develop your system? Well, referencing is one of the few areas where our best advice is learn it and do it. There is absolutely no point in debating it or skipping it. All you will achieve is losing marks for something you must and can master.

What to reference to avoid plagiarism

Students usually ask what to reference and how many references they need in an assignment. As you might expect, there is no set formula to answer this question. We can give you some pointers to develop your referencing skills. First, as you progress in your nursing journey, you will be expected to use more and more evidence. Second, it depends on the nature of the work. If you reflect on your practice, use a case study or have an exam; you will use fewer references at places. Yet the moment you form an opinion about something you need justification or, in other words, evidence, thus reference. Sometimes my colleagues say things like you do not need to prove obvious things like the sky is blue. We would warn you from following such advice, partly because what we call the sky is not a thing, and second, because the colour blue does not exist either. Someone who is blind or lives in the United Kingdom, as opposed to Spain, might have a very different idea of what we mean by blue sky. We rather offer some skills that can help you decide when to reference.

Skills in using evidence and referencing

It is much better to think about referencing like this. Whenever you state something, form an opinion, argue or make a point, ask the following question: how do I know this? I saw it on placement. My lecturer said it in the classroom. The carer of a service user told me. I read a brochure online by the National Autistic Society. I found a research article that compared interventions and also interviewed nurses. These all can be sources and evidence, depending on the nature of your work. How much do you trust them? It is good practice to show different types of evidence. Whilst all these sources can be acceptable, if you only reference grey literature (your lecturer's slide, the National Autistic Society or your placement), your work remains weak. Once you start exploring academic sources, you will be surprised how many things we do that have never been evidenced satisfactorily. One of those things is reflection, which forms a fundamental part of nursing. We know it works, but we hardly have any evidence of why or how (see Chapter 5 about reflection).

How to reference to avoid plagiarism

We have highlighted the importance of using your own words when taking notes, but if you do copy and paste large materials when formulating your assignments, then make sure you highlight these sections, as you have to rewrite them (Morley, 2020). If you do this, you have already done the first step to avoid plagiarism. You rephrased and reworded other people's works. The second step is to acknowledge the source clearly. Do you remember what we said about systems and saving the sources? This is the time that you will need to find all the literature you used, cite it in the main body of your work and provide full details at the end under the heading referencing. Every university tells you which system they use and where to find the guide, so we will not detail it here. There are two major systems that most courses use, Harvard and APA. Some universities will publish their version, usually adding their name to it (Fig. 3.6).

Skills in acknowledging evidence and writing references

There are a few skills that can move your referencing to the highest standards. Make sure you check at least once a year that you are using the latest edition. Download and open the .doc or .pdf document that provides examples. Find the same type of literature such as an edited book and follow their instructions. You must reference it in the text and at the end of the work. Fig. 3.7 shows you the main elements. You need to format the reference list and write it alphabetically. Some sources

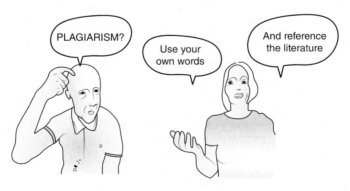

Fig. 3.6   **How to avoid plagiarism.**

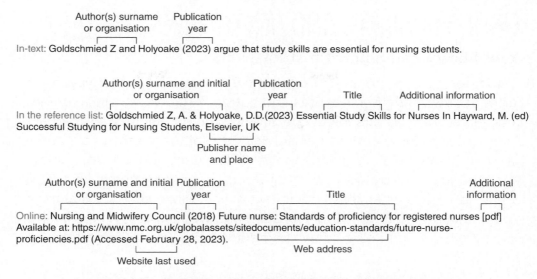

Fig. 3.7 **Example of in-text citation and referencing.**

use the word bibliography and reference interchangeably. In academic terms, they are not the same. The bibliography comes after the reference list and contains materials you accessed and read but did not cite in the main text. Make sure you include every piece of literature you cited in the text in your reference list. You must reference the organisation or person who wrote or published the page and not the web address. For example, the correct reference is National Autistic Society and not autism.org.uk.

TIP

Top 5 tips for effective referencing

1. Know the system your course uses and download the guide.
2. Follow the guide in the text and at the end of the main body.
3. Use software that helps organise and cite your literature.
4. Acknowledge every source you read and used in your work.
5. Always use academic sources in your work wherever you can.

FINAL THOUGHTS AND NEXT STEPS

Your library can help with study skills

It is important to explore your university's library. The earlier you familiarise yourself with their services, the better. You have access to books, articles, reading lists, subject-specific recommendations and tutorials. They publish guides and organise skill development sessions. Your library will have detailed guides to the skills we introduced. Your librarians can support you with which programme your university provides and where you can access additional training. Make sure the first thing you bookmark (save the virtual location and web address) is the library. Pay a visit, create a folder, download guides and watch their tutorials.

NMC

THE NMC SAYS

22.3 'Keep your knowledge and skills up to date, taking part in appropriate and regular learning and professional development activities that aim to maintain and develop your competence and improve your performance'.

A note on technology

You will be reading printed books and articles, using pen and paper and creating handwritten notes and reference lists. However, it is more than likely that many of your activities will have something to do with digital formats. A wide range of assistive and generic digital tools are available to help you if you struggle with some of these study skills or want to make these tasks more interactive. Some tools read out loud a text; others, such as a virtual pacer, can help you focus your eyes and attention (Chapter 2), and of course, there are built-in notepads on all computers. In addition, most universities allow access to a range of free software, and there are many commercial ones. There are programmes that can help create flowcharts, tables or concept maps or organise your literature with the added benefit of creating reference lists. You can check your work for plagiarism (Chapter 6). We want to emphasise how much time and energy you can save if you explore what programmes your university offers for reading, note-taking, literature searching and referencing.

SOCIAL MEDIA

@heblau

'@wenurses explaining to my gran that I teach nursing: "oooh, I didn't realise you needed to study nursing, I thought nurses just knew how'.

Reflect on your learning and study skills. Can you identify one new skill you can learn and practice this week?

_____

_____

_____

_____

TIP

Top 5 things you can do next

1. Save and bookmark your university's library website.
2. Explore all the guides and features your library and course offers.
3. Find out where to ask for help if you struggle with specific skills.
4. Identify your strengths and integrate them into your study skills.
5. Identify the most challenging ideas of this chapter.

CONCLUSION

You have just learnt about four essential study skills that nursing students need to master, and it is a lot to take in. Depending on your age, background, level of education, English language proficiency and digital skills, you will find different parts hard. The trick is to build on your strengths and do more of what you already do well whilst challenging yourself regularly with plans to improve. Like always in life, you will outgrow this introduction, but for now, make sure you get the basics right to excel in your nursing journey.

Now you have finished this chapter. Please make notes on what you have learned.

REFERENCES

APA (2022) *Plagiarism*. Available at: https://apastyle.apa.org/style-grammar-guidelines/citations/plagiarism (Accessed: 29 May 2023).

Buzan, T. (2006). *The Speed Reading Book (new edition): The Revolutionary Approach to Increasing Reading Speed, Comprehension and General Knowledge*. London: BBC Active/Pearson.

Buzan, T. (2011). *Buzan's Study Skills: Mind Maps, Memory Techniques, Speed Reading and More,* London: BBC Active/Pearson.

Goldschmied, A.Z., Zumpalov, L.G. and Holyoake, D.D. (2021). *Two psychiatrists, three boat builders and a million gap hunters: the choices we make in literature.* Available at: https://www.researchgate.net/publication/355844563_Two_psychiatrists_three_boat_builders_and_a_million_gap_hunters_the_choices_we_make_in_literature_reviews (Accessed: 28 February 2023).

Marks-Beale, A. (2002). *Success skills: strategies for study and lifelong learning* (2nd ed.)., Mason, OH: South-Western Educational Publishing

Mental Capacity Act (2005) [online] Available at: https://www.legislation.gov.uk/ukpga/2005/9/contents (Accessed: 28 February 2023).

Morley, J (2020). *Academic phrasebank*. Manchester: The University of Manchester. https://www.phrasebank.manchester.ac.uk/ (Accessed: 28 February 2023).

NICE (2020) *Joint replacement (primary): hip, knee and shoulder* Available at: https://www.nice.org.uk/guidance/ng157 (Accessed: 28 February 2023).

Nursing and Midwifery Council (2018a) *The code*. Available at: https://www.nmc.org.uk/standards/code/ (Accessed: 28 February 2023).

Nursing and Midwifery Council (2018b) *Future nurse: standards of proficiency for registered nurses.* Available at: https://www.nmc.org.uk/globalassets/sitedocuments/education-standards/future-nurse-proficiencies.pdf (Accessed: 28 February 2023)

Paul, R. and Elder, L. (2019). *How to Read a Paragraph: The Art of Close Reading*. London: Rowman and Littlefield.

Rexroth, K. (2023). *Literature. Encyclopaedia Britannica*. Available at: https://www.britannica.com/art/literature. (Accessed: 30 May 2023).

Schöpfel, J. and Farace, D.J. (2015). *"Grey literature"*. In Bates, M.J.; Maack, M.N. (eds.). Encyclopaedia of Library and Information Sciences (3rd ed.). Boca Raton, FL: CRC Press.

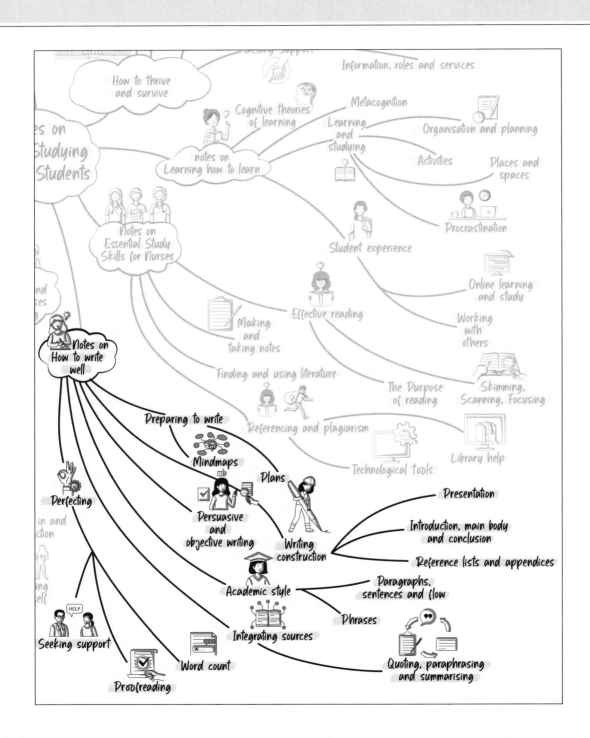

NOTES ON HOW TO WRITE WELL

Rebecca Boden (she/her) ■ Fiona Cust (she/her)
■ Sophie Kempshall (she/her)

INTRODUCTION

It is often a surprise to new nursing students that academic writing is more of a challenge than they expect. For some students, it may have been some time since their formal education, with a long period away from study before starting their nursing programme. Other students may have come recently from studying but still find academic writing challenging, even if they have excelled in their prior studies. However, the good news is that academic writing is a skill to be learned, just like handwashing or any other clinical skill learned throughout the course.

Academic assessments are often unlike exams or coursework that students may have previously experienced in their prior studies, so how would a student expect to instinctively know how to write academically if they haven't had experience studying in higher education? Borglin (2012) states that academic writing differs within professional disciplines. They refer to this as professional socialisation, stating that simply knowing how to write isn't enough to ensure academic success. In essence, this means students must have knowledge of the subject and awareness of the nuances of the profession to write well about it.

Some students may say, 'I'm just not academic enough', when the truth is that they have not yet developed the necessary skills. Your nursing course is likely to be between 2 and 4 years in duration, and in this time, both your nursing knowledge and your academic writing skills will improve.

This chapter will provide you with useful information on numerous areas of academic writing. You will learn how to get started with your writing as well as how to build a persuasive discussion that adheres to the assignment requirements. Moreover, you will learn how to structure your academic writing effectively, ensuring clarity and consistency in your work. Additionally, you will acquire insights into the process of developing a captivating academic argument, as well as be provided with hints and tips that will contribute to your success.

GETTING STARTED

Why is academic writing important?

Academic writing allows students to demonstrate their understanding of module or unit and programme or course learning outcomes, and while most courses will include a range of assessment types, effective academic writing will support many of these assessment strategies. Therefore, succeeding in your course relies on the ability to express your thoughts and ideas effectively to an academic standard.

NMC

THE NMC SAYS

6.1 'Make sure that any information or advice given is evidence based, including information relating to using any health or care products or services'.

Nursing students are developing the ability to deliver evidence-based care, and academic writing is a method which demonstrates your ability to think critically and utilise appropriate evidence. Aveyard et al. (2015) suggest this is an opportunity to challenge your own assumptions and prior knowledge, whilst evaluating the evidence available, to ensure care provided is of the highest standard. The standards of proficiency for registered nurses (NMC, 2018b) also call for nurses to be able to think critically and apply evidence to make informed decisions relating to patient care, and this is a consistent theme that runs through all platforms which comprise the standards.

NMC

THE NMC SAYS

'The confidence and ability to think critically, apply knowledge and skills, and provide expert, evidence-based, direct nursing care therefore lies at the centre of all registered nursing practice'.

Despite the challenges, academic writing can also be immensely rewarding, allowing you to demonstrate the knowledge you have gained related to the subject area.

Preparing to write

Starting to write your assignment can feel overwhelming; however, breaking it into several stages will help the task feel more achievable and will help you plan your time effectively. The earlier you start your assignment plan, the more time you will give yourself to complete your assignment without feeling overwhelmed towards the hand-in date. It is obvious that adhering to hand-in dates is essential, as most universities will not accept late submissions or will have a penalty or grade cap for work submitted after the deadline.

Whilst everyone will find their own ways of working, a common mistake many students make is to rush into the writing phase without the proper preparation. Before you begin, ensure you understand the assignment brief and learning outcomes. The assignment brief outlines the assignment's objective, while the learning outcomes specify the necessary knowledge to complete the assessment, with the requirement that all learning outcomes must be fulfilled to pass. It is then your challenge to identify relevant topics to include which enable you to meet the assignment brief and demonstrate your knowledge aligned to the learning outcomes. Boyd (2014) suggests it is also helpful to review the assignment-marking criteria, as this will provide information on what the marker expects of your work through the various grade points. Chapter 6 discusses some of these points in more detail.

Reading and researching the topic are essential. The more reading you can do related to the topic, the more knowledgeable your argument will be, and this will assist you in writing at the required academic standard.

A good place to start is with the module resources available to you, and from this, you can construct the first stage of your plan.

SOCIAL MEDIA
@NFT_Ian

'Think about the quality of your reading. If you aren't reading high quality stuff it will massively impact on the quality of your writing. Always think about how this impacts on my practice/patient care. Why is something done that way is key to critical analysis'.

Mind maps

Mind maps are a great tool to get started. Sifting through module materials for key topics and themes that link with the assignment brief and module learning outcomes is an excellent way to begin. It allows identification of key points to be included. Initially, these themes may seem somewhat disjointed or even a little chaotic, but this is just a starting point.

As you begin reading, you will find that you can add to your mind map, and as your knowledge of the subject grows, you will be able to make more sense of the ideas you originally included; it may be that you can't include everything you initially wrote on your mind map, but as a result of your reading and research, some ideas will begin to take on more significance than others, allowing you to focus on the most important topics. As well as developing knowledge and understanding the evidence base, reading and researching also allow ideas to be grouped together, which Cottrell (2019) reports can help you form an idea of how you will link themes within your assignment.

Ensuring you are using credible sources of evidence is essential. The internet provides a wealth of information; however, this does not mean it is all accurate and reliable. The purpose of academic writing is to convince the reader of the argument you present, and using stronger, more credible evidence means the reader is more likely to be assured you make a sound argument. Chapter 3 discusses how you can find reliable sources of evidence to support your work.

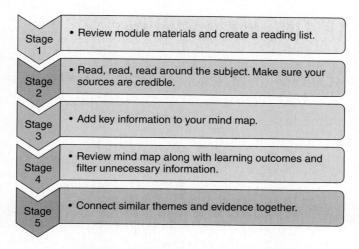

Fig. 4.1   Plan for getting started with a mind map.

Revisit your mind map on a few occasions, or even pin it up on the wall where you can see it (Fig. 4.1).

Essay plan

Once you have devised your mind map, it can be helpful to then organise ideas into a more structured plan. The assignment plan can use bullet points and should demonstrate how themes are grouped together to develop logical progression of ideas. Aveyard et al. (2015) identify the importance of a clear and logical structure in developing a written assignment.

Any assignment plan should be flexible, and you should remain open to change, even once you have begun writing.

SOCIAL MEDIA
@Lucy_uo

'Look at the guidance and split it up into sections to make sure you cover everything. When you are reading, make notes based on those sections—and write where you found them, use quotes if you use the same wording, makes references so much easier'.

CONSTRUCTING YOUR WORK

Different styles of assignments call for different structures and nuances. Table 4.1 provides some examples of how you might change the structure and style of your writing to meet the assignment brief effectively, dependent on the task.

TABLE 4.1 SUGGESTED FORMATS FOR ACADEMIC ASSIGNMENTS

Type of assessment task	Structure and key attributes
Essay	Usually follows the format: • Introduction • Main body • Conclusions • References Typically written in third person. Uses formal language and is concisely written. Based upon research and best available evidence, not the author's own opinion.
Literature review	Literature reviews can be included along with other assignment styles, so it is important to be familiar with the requirements. Structure could include: • Introduction • Methodology—how the literature review was conducted and why this is important • Findings—what did you find out during the literature review? • Conclusion Literature reviews should include appraisal of the quality the evidence included. Formal academic style is required. Written in third person.

TABLE 4.1 SUGGESTED FORMATS FOR ACADEMIC ASSIGNMENTS—cont'd

Type of assessment task	Structure and key attributes
Project or dissertation 	May have several sections, which could include: • Title page • Abstract • Aims and objectives • Literature review • Research methods • Ethical issues • Findings and discussion • Recommendations • References • Appendices Headings can be used to help structure content. Requires a formal academic style, written in third person. Discussion should be concise and well supported with evidence
Reflection 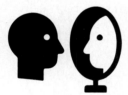	Should be structured according to a defined model such as: Gibbs (1988) • Description • Feelings • Evaluation • Analysis • Conclusion • Action plan Or Driscoll (2007) • What? • So, What? • Now What? Model stages should be used as subheadings to structure assignment. Usually written in first person as a reflection is an exploration of the individual experience. Analysis and Evaluation (Gibbs model) and So What (Driscoll) should comprise much of the word count. Descriptive elements should be kept to the minimum required

Continued

TABLE 4.1 SUGGESTED FORMATS FOR ACADEMIC ASSIGNMENTS—cont'd

Type of assessment task	Structure and key attributes
Report	Reports are often written to present the methods and results from investigations Structure can vary, so ensure you refer to the assignment brief One way you may choose to structure a report is: • Title • Introduction • Methodology • Findings and discussion • Conclusions • Recommendations, if needed • References • Appendices To present information in an easily readable manner, bullet points, use of headings, tables and diagrams can be used. Reports are usually written in third person using formal academic language.

Presentation

Some assignments may call for cover sheets or title pages. This information will be provided by your lecturers, and you should strive to meet these requirements. While it may not be part of the formal marking, this demonstrates quality and attention to detail within your work.

Writing introductions

Introductions usually account for around 10% of the overall word count, and your introduction should clearly identify what the aims of the assignment, as dictated by the learning outcomes, are and how you intend to achieve them. It is also helpful in the introduction to provide additional information to give the reader insight and context for the assignment and to include any relevant definitions to clarify the topic. It can also be beneficial to include information such as how confidentiality has been maintained, if this is relevant, in accordance with the code (NMC, 2018a).

NMC

THE NMC SAYS

5.1 'Respect a person's right to privacy in all aspects of their care'.

Writing the main body

The main body of your work comprises most of your discussion, often around 80%, although this may vary according to the specific style of assignment required. Evidence should be presented to form a logical argument demonstrating a range of ideas and knowledge relating to the assignment brief and learning outcomes. A range of topics will often be discussed to meet the learning outcomes. It is essential for academic writing that this includes citations to the evidence used to inform the argument.

A common misconception students hold is that they must include as many topics as possible to achieve the best grade. This is not true. A skill required in academic writing is to filter out topics which do not add value to your assignment—for example, topics or discussion which does not relate to the assignment brief or module learning outcomes. Using words on irrelevant information limits the words available for the pertinent discussion, leading to a superficial debate. It is often better to include fewer topics (ensuring all learning outcomes are addressed) to allow for deeper exploration of the topics included.

Writing conclusions

Within the conclusions section, you will summarise the key points which you feel represent the strongest argument based on the evidence. The conclusions should not just be a repetition of the earlier discussions. You should not introduce new material into your conclusions, and it is not usually required to include references in this section.

Writing your reference list

Presenting a well-structured and accurate reference list demonstrates your academic skills and it is essential to acknowledge the sources you have used in developing your assignment. Check with your university regarding the required structure for presenting your reference list at the end of your assignment. Please note, your reference list is not included in your word count.

Appendices

Appendix (singular) or appendices (plural) provide additional information to the reader. This additional information tends to be more beneficial in report-style assignments, research assignments or dissertations and may include raw data which is too lengthy to include in the main body of your work. The appendices are included in numerical order after the reference list. Information in the appendices is also not counted in your word limit and is not usually marked (unless the assignment brief specifically states otherwise). The appendices do, however, support the discussion in the main body of your assignment and can demonstrate the quality of your work.

 TIP

- Ensure information in the appendices is relevant.
- Label your appendices—Appendix 1, Appendix 2 and so on.
- Refer to the appendix at relevant points in your discussion, for example, 'see Appendix 1'.
- Ensure you reference the sources of your appendix appropriately.

CASE STUDY

Kiran is a second-year adult nursing student currently studying a registered nurse degree programme. The assessment for the 'Improving Health' module brief is as follows:

Title: The Nurse's Role in Improving Health.

Assignment brief: Write a 2500-word assignment discussing how you will use the nursing process to plan and deliver an episode of health promotion within your chosen area of practice. You should examine the health need, including relevant demographics, public health drivers and a critical analysis of approaches to health promotion in relation to your chosen intervention to ensure your intervention is evidence based.

Module learning outcomes.

1. Critically analyse a range of health promotion strategies.
2. Apply knowledge of demographics, social determinants of health and public health policy to inform health promotion strategies.
3. Demonstrate understanding of the professional requirements of the nurse in relation to health promotion.

As Kiran is on placement with a local health visiting team, Kiran has chosen to focus on reducing infant mortality through the delivery of a safer sleep intervention.

Kiran highlights key points from the assignment brief to assist with structuring the discussion:

Write a 2500-word assignment discussing how you will use the nursing process to plan and deliver an episode of health promotion within your chosen area of practice. You should examine the health need, including relevant demographics and public health drivers and a critical analysis of approaches to health promotion in relation to your chosen intervention to ensure your intervention is evidence based.

Kiran begins by producing the following mind map; they review module sessions and materials such as reading lists for ideas of

Continued

CASE STUDY—cont'd

where to get started with the mind map and then add to it as they begin reading and researching around the subject; see below.

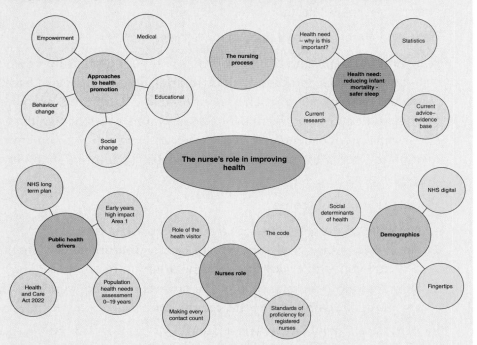

Kiran keeps adding to the mind map until they feel it is comprehensive and then uses the mind map to develop an assignment plan, allowing Kiran to arrange the assignment into a logical format:

Assignment Title	The Nurse's Role in Improving Health
Introduction 250 words	Outline the purpose of the assignment • Nursing process will be used to plan and deliver an episode of health promotion • Use of demographics to identify the public health concern • Identification of public health drivers • Critical analysis of approaches to health promotion • Evidence base

CASE STUDY—cont'd

Assignment Title   The Nurse's Role in Improving Health

Main body 4 × 500 words)	**Theme 1** Introduce the health concern—'infant mortality' (sudden infant death) • Use statistics to identify the scale of concern • Link to social determinants of health • Risk factors • Actions that can be taken to reduce risk, including evidence base **Theme 2** • The intervention: delivery of safer sleep advice during the first post-birth visit • Nursing process • Why use the nursing process? • Use of educational and empowerment approaches to health promotions • Why are these two approaches better suited to the delivery of this intervention? • Why have other approaches to health promotion not been selected (talk about limitations of approaches)? • What is the evidence base for advice given? **Theme 3** • What are the current drivers for improving the health and well-being of children generally: • Health and Care Act 2022 • NHS Long Term Plan • What are the current drivers for improving health and well-being in relation to intervention: • Early years high-impact area 1 • Population health needs 0–19 years **Theme 4** • What is the nurse's role? • NMC expectation linked to the code and standards of proficiency for registered nurses • Making every contact count • Specialist public health nurse/health visitor role • Include evidence on efficacy of nursing interventions in improving health

Continued

CASE STUDY—cont'd

Assignment Title	The Nurse's Role in Improving Health
Conclusions 250 words	Summary of how the proposed intervention aims to improve the health of babies and the importance of the nurse's role in health promotion Summary of challenges identified and how these may be overcome
References	Possible sources of evidence: NHS Digital GOV.UK The Code Standards of proficiency Database search for journal articles and research for: Nurse's role in improving health Nursing process Safer sleep interventions

Once Kiran has completed the assignment plan, they begin writing with one of the themes; it isn't important which one at this stage, as the themes can be rearranged according to the plan later. It can be a hindrance to getting started if you don't feel as confident about the first theme or if you feel you must complete this first; therefore, begin with a theme you feel confident about or interested in, as this will help you to get going.

CRAFTING YOUR ARGUMENT THROUGH OBJECTIVE WRITING

This section of the chapter focuses on crafting persuasive arguments through objective writing, balancing evidence, logical reasoning and critical analysis. By mastering academic writing style techniques, such as the use of academic phrases, quoting, paraphrasing, summarising and structuring sentences and paragraphs, you can ensure readers engage with a strong, well-supported argument that resonates with them.

TIP

Things to consider before you begin...

- Understand the learning objectives of the assignment and refer back to it as you write.
- Review the marking criteria for the academic level that you are writing at.
- Attend any tutorials or supervision sessions that may be available to you.
- Review module materials.
- Avoid leaving things to the last minute.

Constructing your argument

As suggested by Bottomley and Pryjmachuk (2017), an argument involves establishing a claim and then proving your claim using logical, well-considered reasoning that is supported by current evidence-based literature and research. The actual word 'argument' may not appear in your assignment, but arguments and constructive ideas are one of the most important aspects when writing academically. The main aim of academic work is to express a point of view, an opinion on a particular subject, and then to support this with credible evidence and literature.

It is important to have a clear structure to your assignment, as this will help you to express yourself logically and enable the reader to follow the thread of your argument. The skill of providing a clear and articulate argument is a crucial part of the writing process. Organisation is an essential part of building your argument—as discussed earlier, it is helpful to create a plan of your assignment prior to attempting to construct an argument. The layout will help you to clarify both your thinking and your writing process to ensure that your reader can follow the point(s) that you are attempting to make. Remember to offer a clear explanation for each point argued! By doing so, you will demonstrate your credibility which, in turn, will strengthen your argument because the reader will have an understanding as to how you reached your viewpoint.

Where do you begin?

Central to all arguments is a claim, the main point(s) that you are keen to prove (Gimenez, 2018). A strong claim will be interesting, well considered and evidence based. It will certainly be an issue that is worthy of debate! However, you will require proof and justification for your claim; it cannot be your opinion alone. Your proof will be in the form of evidence, data, reliable sources and good examples—all of which must be referenced in the approved style for your institution. It is important to remember at this point that relevant evidence does not necessarily prove a claim, but it does promote a good discussion. There is usually quite a lot of reading and reflecting involved to be in the position to convince your reader that there are justifiable reasons for your claim, for example, why and how the evidence that you are presenting informs your thinking. Be clear, specific and concise.

Where does the argument sit?

It is important, and must become an integral part of your work, to consider and actively seek out alternative points of view and potential objections to the point(s) that you are attempting to claim. It is human nature to be drawn into ideas that support our own ways of thinking, called biases; this can result in a narrow or flawed argument. Hopkins and Reid (2018) suggest that by deliberately engaging with objections and weaving them into our own way of thinking (our inbuilt biases), we can develop a more nuanced and rounded argument.

Read widely around the point that you are trying to make or prove—provide debate and discussion. Seek out literature that neither proves nor disproves your claim to ensure that the evidence you are citing is not one-sided. It's almost as if you are having an argument within your writing, and it makes it very interesting for your reader. Bring your discussion to life! If you can provide a cohesive discussion within your writing that is well evidenced and has explored all angles to your claim (not just your own), you may be able to 'persuade' your reader to explore your argument in more detail or even join you in your way of thinking. The strength of your evidence can make or break your argument, so choose carefully and use it wisely.

When you are writing your conclusion, you should aim to present a balanced summary of your argument. Choose your wording and language carefully to enhance the strength of your findings. You may be able to take the opportunity to make some recommendations too, for example, improve practice and to identify future openings and collaborations for further research.

TIP

When including evidence:

- Read widely and support your claim with evidence from credible, academic sources, BUT be open to interpretation.
- Structure is important—keep the flow of your assignment logical and ordered. Be clear, specific and concise.
- Be careful with logical fallacies! Just because there is evidence does not automatically prove an argument. It is important to explain how, and why, your evidence is credible, valid and sufficient.
- Embrace opposing viewpoints. Use them wisely to provide interesting discussion and debate. Provide evidence that you have considered all potential counterarguments.

Academic writing style

Producing written work as part of an exam, essay, dissertation or another form of assessment requires an approach to organisation and use of language and structure. When writing academically, there is a process involved which includes reading, finding and evaluating information, editing and proofreading your work and reflecting on any feedback that may have been provided to you.

Academic writing can be conventional, flexible and adaptable. When you are tasked with an assignment and learning outcomes to be demonstrated within the assignment, it is not the point for you and your peers to produce exactly the same work but to provide a shared framework with different visions, ideas and concepts. Academic writing uses more formal terminology than everyday communication. It is important NOT to write as you speak but to hit the right level of formality within your work.

Formal language

Briefly, academic writing often uses fewer words to help you develop a more concise style of writing. This also helps with maintaining your word limitation.

For example:

- Talk about—discuss
- To finish—conclude
- Carry out—perform

Academic writing tends to avoid the types of abbreviations used in day-to-day speak, known as contractions. The words are usually written out in full. It is important to avoid a style of writing that is conversational (colloquial). When writing academically, colloquialisms should be avoided and replaced with a more formal, professional style.

Examples of how to avoid contractions:

- You're—you are
- Isn't—is not
- Aren't—are not
- Can't—cannot
- Doesn't—does not

If you are using an abbreviation, use the full form of the abbreviated name/reference in the first instance, including the abbreviation in brackets. When you use it after this within your writing, you can use just the abbreviation.

For example:

- Nursing Midwifery Council (NMC)
- Royal College of Nursing (RCN)
- Heart rate (HR)
- Blood pressure (BP)

WRITING OBJECTIVELY

Although you may already have an opinion or theory that you are keen to get across within your writing, it is important that, to build a compelling objective case, you support your ideas and statements using credible evidence and data (Price, 2021). All sources used and mentioned in your work must be referenced correctly using the system recommended by your university (Table 4.2).

TIP

When writing academically:

- It is usually better to avoid using the first person (I or we). The first person is commonly used if you are putting forward your own informed opinion—for example, as part of a reflection or a discussion section.
- Try to avoid adjectives that imply a value judgement, for example, 'fantastic, amazing, brilliant, rubbish, boring'.
- Avoid using cliched phrases, for example, 'at the end of the day...' 'the flip side...', 'as a matter of fact....' 'to be honest....'
- Try not to overstate within your writing—extremely, definitely, the most, the least, always, never, loads...
- Avoid writing as you would speak (conversational or casual writing): focus upon a more analytical, professional style (academic writing).

TABLE 4.2 SOURCES OF EVIDENCE

Primary sources

- Include any information or data that you have found, collected or generated to illustrate your argument or to explore your ideas/hypotheses. Primary sources include texts that you are analysing, survey responses, interviews, experimental data, artefacts, etc.

Secondary sources

- Should be used to build a strong foundation of background thinking, ideas and theories. This will strengthen and help to validate the point/idea that you are trying to make. Secondary sources include books, published research, journals, presentations, films, audio recordings, etc.

Sentence structure, paragraphs and flow of writing

To effectively write a paragraph, you must first think about sentence structure. An effective sentence should have a subject or purpose and include a complete thought, which is sometimes considered a clause. Some sentences may contain more than one clause which may or may not be related. Avoid simple sentences such as 'research was done', as this can make your work difficult to read; instead, use a conjunction or punctuation to join sentences such as 'Research was undertaken, but the findings were inconclusive'.

In academic writing, there are two primary voices: active and passive. The active voice is preferred, as it engages the reader, provides clarity and conciseness and emphasises the subject performing an action. For instance, one can write 'The nurse completed the patient observation' or even 'I completed the patient observations.' On the other hand, the passive voice is commonly used in nursing to establish an objective tone. Sentences in passive voice shift the focus to the object or action being performed. For example, one might say 'The patient had their observation taken by the nurse'. Depending on the nature of your assignment, it is crucial to be aware and proficient in both writing styles.

 TIP

Remember when formulating sentences:

- All sentences should begin with a capital letter and end with a suitable punctuation, such as a full stop or question mark.
- Don't write overly long sentences (sometimes called 'run-on'); they can make your work difficult to read.
- Avoid short or fragmented sentences.
- Make sure your sentence has a purpose.
- Don't open a sentence with 'because' or 'and'.

Paragraphs are the building blocks of your written work and will contain a number of sentences to develop depth or argument as discussed. A good assignment will organise the content clearly and coherently within

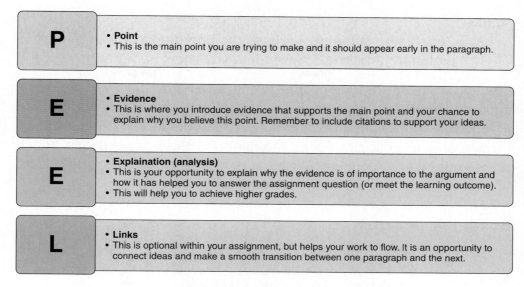

Fig. 4.2   PEEL model of paragraph structure.

paragraphs. When writing academically, this can be difficult, as there may be a complexity of ideas that you are working with. However, paragraphs make it easier for the reader to follow your writing, and, often, the assignment appears to be more logical in structure.

The PEEL model (University of Hull, 2023) is a well-known and useful technique to help you structure your paragraphs (Fig. 4.2).

Here is an example of how to structure a paragraph:

Point

- The first sentence (topic sentence) states the main idea or area to be covered by the paragraph.
- An explanation or a definition can be used to clarify any difficult or unfamiliar terminology that has been introduced in the first sentence.

Evidence

- One or more sentences introducing key ideas, quotes, evidence or data.

Explanation

- Explores what the evidence means, how it can be summarised or/and whether it needs to be challenged.

Links

- Concluding sentence—relates the paragraph to your overall argument and links forward into your next paragraph.

It is important to remember that the final sentence is often the most important part of a paragraph, as it clarifies your understanding and identifies how it contributes to your overall argument. A paragraph will usually only discuss one idea as outlined in the first sentence (topic/ point sentence). If your paragraph is drifting away from this first idea, then you need to split it into more than one paragraph.

Academic phrases

Offering alternative viewpoints or presenting differing findings can often be challenging for new academic writers; however, there are many academic phrases that are extensively used to smoothly transition into the discussion of an alternate point of view (The University of Manchester, 2023). Presenting a balanced discussion is important in your work. We often hold beliefs and opinions that are influenced by our experiences; however, when we delve deeper into the research, it becomes impossible to discount the literature that challenges our preexisting opinions. However, many inexperienced writers will do exactly that, which quite often results in a descriptive, inaccurate and biased assignment. Table 4.3 provides some useful phrases that you can use within your work.

Think about assignments you may have written in the past; did you search for information that supported your original belief? Did you discount evidence that disagreed with your argument? How did you carry out your search? How did you determine where to find your evidence? How did you start your literature search?

_____

_____

_____

_____

_____

TABLE 4.3 USEFUL PHRASES THAT CAN BE USED WITHIN YOUR WORK

Phrases	When to use them
However, furthermore, in addition	Support the flow of your writing or to expand the information that you are including, e.g., 'furthermore, author (date) suggested that...'
Interestingly, similarly, comparably, likewise	To link sources that support each other, e.g., 'similarly, author (date) reported....'
Noticeably, conversely, in contrast to, on the contrary	Compare and contrast findings from various sources related to the same topic, e.g., 'this is in contrast to findings reported by author (date)...'
Significantly, noticeably, notable, noteworthy	To draw attention to findings, e.g., 'a notable finding of this study....'
Reported, stated, found that, claimed, suggested	When discussing what an author has written within your work; 'author (date) suggested that XXX'
Thus far, to conclude, in summary	When drawing a section to a close or within the concluding paragraph

Specifically seeking out information that supports your own ideas is recognised as confirmation bias; this includes ignoring information that contradicts your own beliefs (Acks, 2019). So, when you are planning your argument(s) for your first or next assignment, be aware of how your own behaviours are influencing the information that you are choosing to include in your discussion. You should search for literature on a topic and use this to inform your writing, not the other way round!

INTEGRATING SOURCES

What is the difference between quoting, paraphrasing and summarising?

Understanding the various methods of incorporating external sources into your writing is essential for effective and credible communication.

TABLE 4.4 ACADEMIC TERMINOLOGY

Quoting—directly including within your writing, the published words or data you have found in a source.

Paraphrasing—expressing, but in your own words, the arguments, ideas or other material that you have found published elsewhere.

Paraquoting—paraphrasing an idea but retaining a few important words or phrases from the original article/book in quotation marks.

Summarising—providing a coherent overview of a single larger area of work or multiple sources.

It is an essential and necessary part of your work to quote/paraphrase, but it is important to demonstrate your understanding and knowledge of what you are actually writing about. Skilful use of sources are important elements of the critical writing process.

In basic terms, paraphrasing is reading something and then rewriting the information in your own words. Through this process, you are not simply copying what somebody else has said, you are demonstrating your understanding of the information that is being conveyed (Staffordshire University, 2023). Whereas using a direct quote is writing it exactly as the original author did, use speech marks to identify it as a quote (see Table 4.4). In both cases, you must cite the author of the original source of information, using the required referencing approach. When writing academically, you need to support the statements you are making with evidence from what other people have written about. You must demonstrate that you have explored the theory that underpins the topic that you are discussing.

Examples of using direct quotes and paraphrasing:

- **A direct quote: speech marks have been used and the author and page number has been cited:**
  The NMC (2018a, p 4) states that 'nurses, midwives and nursing associates uphold the code within the limits of their competence. This means, for example, that while a nurse and nursing associate will play different roles in an aspect of care, they will both uphold the standards in the code within the contribution

they make to overall care. The professional commitment to work within one's competence is a key underpinning principle of the code (see section 13) which, given the significance of its impact on public protection, should be upheld at all times'.

- **This could be paraphrased to:**
  Nurses have a responsibility to ensure that they are competent when delivering care; the NMC (2018a) outlines professional standards that their regulated professionals are required to uphold, with emphasis being placed on recognising professional limitations by working within their scope of practice.

Knowing when to quote and when to paraphrase is crucial in academic writing. Direct quotes are used when a formal definition is required, emphasising specific language as paramount. They are also employed when quoting an opinion, regardless of personal agreement, or when reporting direct speech to capture the reactions or experiences of individuals involved. Additionally, direct quotes can be useful in highlighting specific features of the author's writing style. However, it is essential to exercise caution in using direct quotes, as their overuse can diminish the demonstration of understanding. On the other hand, paraphrasing is employed to elaborate on or clarify concepts and definitions. It serves as a tool for critical engagement with opinions or sources, allowing you to demonstrate your comprehension. Paraphrasing is also effective for summarising the reactions or experiences of one or more individuals, particularly when the general concept takes precedence over the specific language being used.

 TIP

For effective paraphrasing:

- Read the source—you need to make sure that you fully understand what the author is stating. You might find it useful to make notes as you are reading.
- Rewrite the information using your own words—you are summarising what the author has said; this demonstrates your understanding.

Continued

TIP—cont'd

- Be concise; do not overcomplicate the point that you are trying to make.
- Paraphrasing provides the opportunity to make links to other sources of information, allowing you to 'compare and contrast' what different authors have reported.
- Avoid using synonyms to change the occasional word within the original sentence. If you maintain the original sentence structure and merely change a few words, you are not paraphrasing.
- Use a similarity checker prior to submitting your work; this will identify ineffective paraphrasing within your work.
- Always cite the author(s)!

PERFECTING YOUR WRITING

The last section of the chapter discusses three key aspects for refining your work: word counts, proofreading and seeking support. Word counts help manage requirements, proofreading enhances clarity and accuracy and seeking support encourages the utilisation of available resources to strengthen your writing and ensure overall quality.

Word counts

Writing to a word count

Word counts are part of the challenge of academic writing for several reasons:

- The word count provides an indication of the level of detail and depth you should go into.
- To ensure parity, the student has the same number of words as their peers.
- To test your ability to write academically, being able to maintain within a word count requires a concise writing style.
- To demonstrate your critical analytical skills to stay within a word count, you need to focus upon the key points that you are trying to make; this puts critical thinking into practice.

Going over a word count

There is usually a discretionary allowance of 10% over the word allowance or 10% under, without grade penalties being awarded. But ensure that you confirm this with your tutor or lecturer. To try to avoid going over the word count (or under), consider the following:

- Do you have a clear plan, and have you stuck to it?
- Are you selective with your arguments and points of discussion? What is your mission statement or key argument, and how does each section help you to form this?
- Waffling (!)—using 200 words when 100 will do. Aim to work on developing a concise academic writing style, as discussed earlier.

TIP

Sticking to the word count:

- Plan what key points you want to make and what percentage of your word count you are going to spend on each.
- Avoid repeating arguments or points of discussion. If you have highlighted a point, then move on to your next one. There is no need for reiteration.
- Are any of your paragraphs making the same point? Could you link them?
- Rather than trying to demonstrate all the reading that you may have done, be selective and focus upon the most important and relevant materials. Explain why you have chosen them specifically.
- Remember to be concise; this allows more words to use on things that are important, for example, critical analysis and discussion.

Proofreading your work before submission

Proofreading your work allows you to identify errors and gives you the opportunity to correct them before submission. It is not just an effective method of scanning for grammatical or spelling errors, it provides the opportunity to review sentence structure and meaning. Sometimes when constructing assignments, our thoughts are occurring more quickly than our fingers can type or write! This can sometimes lead to assignments not flowing efficiently or the meaning to become lost within a long, rambling sentence. Remember to write concisely!

A useful approach is reading your work with a fixed purpose. For example, reading your work through with the sole purpose of checking that all references are present, correct and in the right format. Then, you might read it through again with the purpose of checking for correct spelling. Above all else, you need to give yourself time to proofread your work.

TIP

Proofreading:

- **Give yourself enough time.**
- **Read it out loud; there are numerous useful digital tools that will do this for you. This method is an effective way of seeing if your work makes sense.**
- **You may find it useful to print a copy of your reference list out; as you proofread your assignment, highlight or tick them off the reference list. This is an effective way of identifying sources that you may have missed.**
- **Proofread your work with a specific purpose.**

SOCIAL MEDIA
@VirtueKarin

'Have someone nonmedical who is happy to read your work. They may not understand the context, but they will understand if it reads well'.

Over to you... proofread the paragraph below; how many errors can you identify? What type of assessment might this be?

_____

_____

_____

_____

_____

"Reflecting upon practice provides the oportunity for practitioners to review event's and use the outcomes to enhance future practice (*REF). This idea is supported by Dewey (1933) who argued that reflection allows individualz to inform future action through the analysis of an experience. as a nurse reflective practice is embedded within my role, therefore becoming a reflective teacher has been a wee natural transition. Although Rogers (5010) suggested that reflection is a process that is usually prompted by an unsatisfactory outcome, that is not always the case in nursing. Healthcare professionals are encouraged to reflex on positive experiences as well, for the same purpose of researching evidence to understand the event and use this knowledge to inform future practice. Harrison (2018) identified that learning and development is influenced by our existing values, beliefs, and experiense. I have totally found it useful complete reflections on like both positive and negative incidences during my professional development."

How did you get on? There are, in fact, 10 errors, which range from spelling to the use of a colloquialism. What about the last sentence? Do you think it is appropriate to include 'totally' and 'like' in this way within your academic work? Using a conversational approach within academic work is often inappropriate, so when you are proofreading your work, be mindful of the tone that you are using, as discussed earlier in the chapter.

If you identified this to be a reflective assignment, well done! Notice that 'I' is used within the example. It is important to understand whether it is appropriate to write in the 'first' person, as most academic pieces of work will identify a 'third'-person approach. Remember, as mentioned previously, an exception to the rule is reflective practice because you are discussing your experience and how you have/will continue to develop your professional practice. Always ask if you are unsure which style you are expected to be writing in.

Seeking support

We all need help and support sometimes; the most important thing is recognising when and where to appropriately seek it from. Refer back to Chapter 1, which outlined some of the people who may be able to support you; refer to Chapter 6 for information about specific help for assessments. We all learn differently; therefore, it makes sense that we all face different challenges at various times within our academic and personal journeys. If you are unsure of what support you can access, then ASK!

What are your own challenges? What support do you have access to?

_____

_____

_____

_____

_____

Take this along with you to your next tutorial as a prompt for discussion.

SOCIAL MEDIA
bgpink00
'Get help from library staff, proofread and proofread and read again'.

Remember to use your feedback (see Chapter 6). When your assignment is marked, the person marking your submission will have provided comments on how to improve your work. Do not take this as a criticism; there is always room for improvement. Sometimes we refer to these suggestions as 'feed forward'. As you move through your course, the academic expectations increase, so use the feedback/feedforward as stepping stones to develop your academic writing skills.

CONCLUSION

This chapter has, hopefully, provided some key tips and guidance for writing an academic assignment. Academic writing is a skill that will evolve over time with both practice and experience. It is very important to review and learn from the feedback that you receive from your tutors and lecturers too.

Several key points to remember before you even begin to put pen to paper:

Plan your assignment carefully; create a mind map as demonstrated earlier in the chapter if you find this helpful. Think about the structure of your assignment, and allocate your word count to each section to ensure that you remain within your word count. What are the learning outcomes? Highlight them! Throughout the entirety of writing, revisit your learning outcomes regularly and question whether you are addressing them. Cross-reference consistently; have them by your side as you write.

Read widely! Source your materials and evidence from reliable and credible journals, books and articles. Before you begin your assignment, if you have a good knowledge base around the subject you are writing about, the flow will be a lot easier. The importance of prereading, planning and rereading cannot be underestimated.

Utilise the support available—your tutors, lecturers, library staff and academic support/study skills teams. Attend tutorials; they are there to guide you and you can ask specific questions related to your subject area. It is your opportunity to clarify points and 'clear' your thought processes a little.

Allow time. Last-minute, thrown-together assignments rarely do well and cause unnecessary stress and anxiety. Plan, plan, read and read. But allow yourself time to do so. Feeling time pressured and rushed will increase your stress levels considerably.

Try to remain on point. Reread your work carefully and at regular intervals. Ask someone to proofread for you. Check your grammar, punctuation and spelling. Does it make sense? Are you making your point clear and concisely? Can the reader follow what you are trying to say?

Finally, your references. Have you referenced correctly within your writing, and are they referenced correctly in your reference list? If you have copied and pasted a link, click on it and ensure that it works AND it takes you to where you want to go.

Breathe. If you are well prepared, have read widely and taken time with your writing; this will be demonstrated within both your work and the grade and feedback awarded.

Now you have finished this chapter. Please make notes on what you have learned.

_____

_____

_____

_____

_____

_____

_____

_____

_____

_____

_____

_____

_____

REFERENCES

Acks, A. (2019) *The bubble of confirmation bias*. New York: Enslow Publishing.

Aveyard, H., Sharp, P. and Woolliams, M. (2015) *A beginner's guide to critical thinking and writing in health and social care*. Second edition. Maidenhead: McGraw-Hill

Borglin, G. (2012) 'Promoting critical thinking and academic writing skills in nurse education'. *Nurse Education Today* (32) pp. 611–613.

Bottomley, J. and Pryjmachuk, S. (2017) *Academic Writing and Referencing for your Nursing Degree (Critical Study Skills)*. St Albans: Critical Publishing.

Boyd, C. (2014) *Study skills for nurses*. Hoboken: Wiley.

Cottrell, S. (2019) *The Study Skills Handbook*. London: Macmillan Education.

Driscoll, J.J. (2007) 'Supported reflective learning: the essence of clinical supervision?' Chapter 2 in *Practising Clinical Supervision: A Reflective Approach for Healthcare Professionals* (2nd edition). London: Bailliere Tindall. pp. 27–50.

Gibbs, G. (1988) *Learning by doing: A guide to teaching and learning methods*. Oxford: Further Education Unit Oxford Polytechnic.

Gimenez, J. (2018) *Writing for Nursing and Midwifery Students*. London: Palgrave Macmillan.

Hopkins, D. and Reid, T. (2018) *The Academic Skills Handbook: Your Guide to Success in Writing, Thinking and Communicating at University*. First Edition. London: Sage.

Nursing and Midwifery Council (2018a) *The Code: Professional standards of behaviour for nurses, midwives and nursing associates*. Available at: https://www.nmc.org.uk/standards/code/ (Accessed: 22 February 2023).

Nursing and Midwifery Council (2018b) *Standards of proficiency for registered nurses*. Available at: https://www.nmc.org.uk/globalassets/sitedocuments/standards-of-proficiency/nurses/future-nurse-proficiencies.pdf (Accessed: 22 February 2023).

Price, B (2021) *Critical Thinking and Writing in Nursing. Transforming Nursing Practice Series*. 5th Edition. London: Sage.

Staffordshire University (2023) *Study skills*. Available at: https://libguides.staffs.ac.uk/study-skills (Accessed: 22 February 2023).

The University of Manchester (2023) *Academic Phrasebank*. Available at https://www.phrasebank.manchester.ac.uk/. (Accessed: 22 February 2023).

University of Hull (2023) *Grammar resource: Paragraph structure*. Available at: https://libguides.hull.ac.uk/writing/paras (Accessed: 22 February 2023).

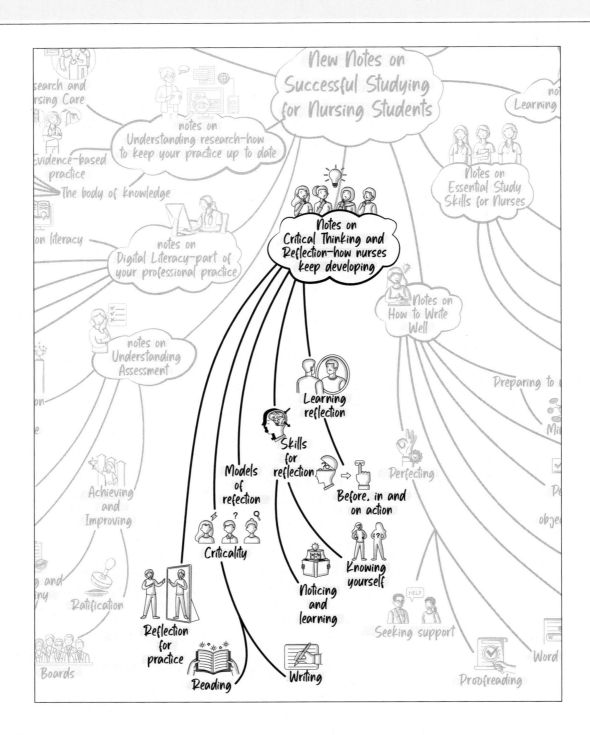

5

NOTES ON CRITICAL THINKING AND REFLECTION—HOW NURSES KEEP DEVELOPING

Debbie Roberts (she/her) ■ **Victoria Carter (she/her)**

INTRODUCTION

This chapter will delve into the crucial concepts of reflection and critical thinking, equipping you with practical tips to excel as a nursing student. Starting with clear definitions of reflection, we'll establish its significance in the learning journey of a nurse and its practical application in nursing practice. Throughout the chapter, we'll provide hints and tips to guide you in reflecting before, during and after taking action, ultimately boosting your confidence as an emerging nursing student and future registrant. To help you structure your thoughts during reflection, we'll present several models of reflection. Additionally, as reflective writing often forms an integral part of nursing education, we'll share ideas that foster critical reading, thinking and writing. This approach will enable you to question and learn from both the literature you encounter and your experiences in nursing practice. Towards the end of the chapter, we'll encourage you to consider developing action points, showcasing how you actively use reflection as a powerful tool for learning on your educational journey. By embracing reflection and critical thinking, you'll enhance your capabilities as a nursing student, setting a strong foundation for your future career in healthcare.

WHAT IS REFLECTION IN NURSING?

This first part of the chapter will introduce the concept of reflection and its application in both nurse education and in nursing practice. Our goal is to provide you with a deeper understanding of reflection and to encourage you to start incorporating it into your learning process. Furthermore, we'll highlight the connections between reflection and critical thinking, laying the foundation for your journey towards becoming a registered nurse.

So, let's start by examining what is meant by reflection. There are many definitions of reflection, and some are more helpful to nursing students than others. You may have already come across the term reflection or reflective practice. If so, start to write down some ideas about what it means to you. (There are no right or wrong answers to this exercise: it's just to get you thinking.)

What does the term 'reflection' or 'reflective practice' mean to you?

_____

_____

_____

_____

_____

You might find it helpful to look at some dictionary definitions to compare your notes to.

Dictionary definitions describe some options for the literal translation and meaning of reflection; however, none of them specifically mentions reflection as a tool for learning or nursing, so the dictionary definitions are not really helpful in terms of what it means in a nursing context.

Perhaps the most famous writer on reflection is Schon (1987, p26). He describes two forms of reflection and provides the following definitions:

Reflection in action:	Reflection on action:
'Where we may reflect in the midst of action without interrupting it. Our thinking serves to reshape what we are doing while we are doing it'.	'Thinking back on what we have done in order to discover how our knowing in action may have contributed to an unexpected outcome. We may do so after the fact in tranquillity, or we may pause in the midst of action (stop and think)'.

These definitions refer to learning in a professional context, although they are not specifically about learning in nursing. Schon (1987) is writing about how professionals (particularly those from practice-based disciplines) learn from their experiences. His definitions suggest that, as a professional, it is possible to reflect whilst you are undertaking a nursing intervention (in action) and also, a slower and deliberate reflection that takes place after a nursing intervention is complete (on action).

The following definition by Howatson-Jones (2010, p6) is perhaps more helpful because it relates to learning for nursing:

'Reflection is a way of examining your experience in order to look for the possibility of other explanations and alternative approaches to doing things. It may happen as part of an activity or when you have more time to think about what you have experienced'.

Price and Harrington (2010, p25) expand on this and define reflection as:

'A process whereby experience is examined in ways that give meaning to interaction...[it] engages the emotions as well as reasoning, reflection needs to take account of the feelings engendered within an interaction and to allow that perceptions (how we interpret matters) may sometimes prove erroneous. While reflection is most closely associated with human interactions and especially clinical events, it is not limited to these. We may, for instance, reflect upon the written accounts of experiences, such as those shared by dying patients. Reflection may be used in the service of different nursing goals- those that are designed to tell us something about how we think, what we value and with regard to ways in which practice could be improved'.

You can see from the definitions offered by Howatson-Jones (2010) and Price and Harrington (2010) that reflection is about learning from experience and it is possible to reflect on incidents that take place in practice involving yourself and others, and it is also possible to reflect on written accounts of patient stories or clinical case studies or medical records. In all cases, reflection is about learning.

Reflection and critical thinking in nurse education are closely linked. Thinking critically also takes conscious effort and practice because it is concerned with what has been learned and how it has been learned. It involves judgement and decision-making.

NMC

THE NMC SAYS

'The confidence and ability to think critically, apply knowledge and skills, and provide expert, evidence-based, direct nursing care therefore lies at the centre of all registered nursing practice'.

As a registered nurse, you are expected to draw on theoretical and practical knowledge and be aware of your limitations. In order to make decisions, you will need to show that you have highly developed skills of critical analysis. Reflection is one mechanism to enhance your critical thinking skills (Jasper, 2013).

Having looked at some definitions of reflection and considered the need for nurses to learn from their experiences; this next section of the chapter will help you to get started with reflection.

LEARNING TO REFLECT

Reflection is an essential aspect of all of our lives. We have an experience, we think about why we reacted in a certain way and we then consider whether we need to take action and alter our response to similar experiences in the future. The human species has continued to survive across the millennia by effectively using this process (Murdoch-Eaton and Sandars, 2014). So, it is useful to think of reflection as a way in which professionals learn from experience. Learning from experience (and therefore learning through reflection) is about learning by doing. As a learner, only you can reflect on your own experiences, and so, the learning is personal to you. Educators can intervene in various ways to assist, but they only have access to your thoughts and feelings through what you choose to reveal. As a learner, you are in control.

Reflection necessarily involves learning about yourself and is associated with deeper learning. This means being honest with yourself when examining what took place during an event. You may need to explore and challenge your attitudes and values as well as your approach to care. So, sometimes, reflection can be an uncomfortable activity. Learning to reflect as a future nurse is more than just thinking things over: a change of perspective and subsequent behaviour is required. The process enables you to start to think about what might have happened if you had acted differently. The process also enables you to pinpoint why certain nursing encounters went well, so you can reproduce those actions in other similar circumstances as you meet them during your career. See Fig. 5.1 for the five key elements of reflection.

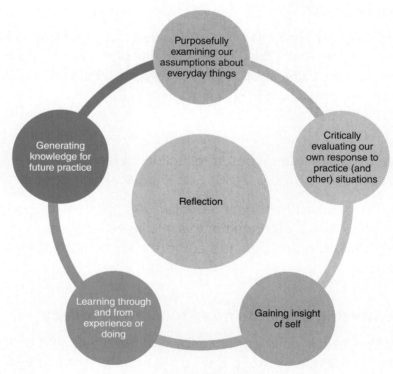

Fig. 5.1   Elements of reflection.

Here are some nursing Tweets about experiences of reflection; note how many of the five aspects from Fig. 5.1 you can identify from these Tweets.

SOCIAL MEDIA

@melhayward

'we're interested in 'positive reflection' rather than 'negative reflection' too often it's used to unpick issues & difficulties. It's not used enough to understand & amplify; celebrate good practice'.

@CNENetworkUK

'Lots of reflection through studying and formal essays, but also much more Reflection happens naturally just thinking about practice. It's used to feel forced but actually it's so important, healthy and happens without realising it'.

@CiaraMoloney5

'I do it every day and this constant thinking can get exhausting at times... ?? BUT. There have been experiences in practice - nursing and education - where reflection has been so helpful for mentalising... as well as being kinder to myself'.

Generally, there are three types of reflection: before action, in action and on action (Nicol and Dosser, 2016). See Fig. 5.2, which describes these.

You may be required to submit reflective assignments as part of your preregistration nurse programme: this will involve reflecting on action. There are some top tips from the authors about reflective writing later in the chapter.

Why do nursing students need to learn to reflect?

Learning to reflect is an important aspect of becoming and being a registered nurse. All nurses in the United Kingdom are bound by the code

Reflection before action
Involves thinking about what you aim to achieve and understanding the means by which this will be accomplished, and this may include drawing on previous experience.

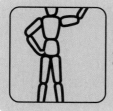

Reflection in action
Relates to your conduct while undertaking the task and allows you to modify what you are doing while you are doing it. This is a fastpaced activity and one where you do not stop to think. This is commonly described as 'thinking on your feet'.

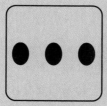

Reflection on action
Involves looking retrospectively at how practice was executed and analysing the information gathered in terms of knowledge, new learning and professional development (Schon 1983; Rolfe et al., 2010). It requires us to create new habits. It requires us to pause (often in silence) and resist the urge to respond immediately, it is slow and deliberate, and requires practice to gain mastery.

Fig. 5.2   Three types of reflection.

(NMC, 2018b, p5), which 'contains a series of statements that taken together signify what good practice by nurses, midwives and nursing associates looks like. It puts the interests of patients and service users first, is safe and effective, and promotes trust through professionalism'. Once registered, you will be expected to demonstrate that you continuously adhere to the code (NMC, 2018b) in every aspect of the work you are required to undertake. It is central to revalidation, the process every nurse must regularly complete to remain on the register as a nurse and is used as a focus for professional reflection. Therefore, reflection is a skill that you will use throughout your career as a nurse.

According to Schon (1983) becoming an effective reflective practitioner is the difference between effective and ineffective practice; see Table 5.1.

TABLE 5.1 SCHON (1983) EFFECTIVE AND INEFFECTIVE PRACTITIONER TRAITS

Effective practitioner	Ineffective practitioner
Is able to recognise and explore confusing or unique (positive or negative) events that occur during practice.	Is confined to repetitive and routine practice, neglecting opportunities to think about what they are doing.

The NMC (2018a) standards of proficiency for registered nurses, under which all preregistration nurse education programmes are governed in the United Kingdom, are grouped into seven areas of nursing, known as 'platforms'. Platform 1, 'being an accountable professional', also reinforces the importance of being able to learn from experience.

NMC

THE NMC SAYS

'Registered nurses continually reflect on their practice and keep abreast of new and emerging developments in nursing, health and care'.

As a nursing student, you will be expected to learn from your experiences in both university and placement. You can use your experience when things went well and also draw on aspects where things did not go so well in order to learn from them. Both are equally important.

GETTING STARTED WITH SKILLS FOR REFLECTION

Here, the chapter describes reflecting before, during and after action. This section of the chapter may be particularly helpful to read before you have your first placement. It explores reflecting beforehand (anticipatory reflection) and why this is so important for beginning students (reflecting during action and after action).

Knowing yourself

Nursing is an emotional endeavour; as nurses, we meet people when they are at their most vulnerable. There will undoubtedly be times where you will feel uncomfortable or vulnerable; there will be times of self-doubt, distrust and anxiety. It is important to understand our personal values and beliefs to become self-aware, and this requires a conscious process to know what makes us feel and act the way we do.

How do you feel about the following:

- Caring for a person who is a prisoner.
- Caring for a person seeking abortion.
- Caring for someone who may become an organ donor.
- Responding to a family who asks you not to tell their loved one that they have a terminal diagnosis and will die.

_____

_____

_____

_____

_____

The code (NMC, 2018b) has several statements that should be considered in relation to your personal views, beliefs and values. It is important to think about what you believe in order to care for others in a professional, caring manner.

NMC

THE NMC SAYS

You make sure that those receiving care are treated with respect, that their rights are upheld and that any discriminatory attitudes and behaviours towards those receiving care are challenged.

4.4 'Tell colleagues, your manager and the person receiving care if you have a conscientious objection to a particular procedure and arrange for a suitably qualified colleague to take over responsibility for that person's care'.

20.2 'Act with honesty and integrity at all times, treating people fairly and without discrimination, bullying or harassment'.

20.5 'Treat people in a way that does not take advantage of their vulnerability or cause them upset or distress'.

20.6 'Stay objective and have clear professional boundaries at all times with people in your care (including those who have been in your care in the past), their families and carers'.

20.7 'Make sure you do not express your personal beliefs (including political, religious or moral beliefs) to people in an inappropriate way'.

With reference to the NMC code (2018b) excerpts, start to think about your beliefs and values and what these might mean in terms of being able to uphold the code. What are your assumptions? And where do your beliefs come from?

_____

_____

_____

_____

_____

Lucy (2012) writes an interesting reflection from their perspective as a nursing student when they were allocated a placement learning opportunity with custody nurses in a police station. In the reflection, Lucy (2012) describes how the experience challenged their preconceived ideas. Moreover, they outline plans and strategies to handle similar situations in the future. You may like to search for this article in your University library. You will find the reference in the reference list.

Before action

One technique for starting to reflect before undertaking any nursing activity is known as anticipatory reflection (Van Manen, 1991). Starting to reflect before going into practice or before undertaking a specific intervention, such as administering medication under supervision, can be particularly helpful for novice students. You can start to think about what you might see, hear, say, feel and more. You can start to prepare for the experience so that you can make the most of every learning opportunity.

 Let's imagine you have just received your first placement allocation and you will be attending a nursing home to care for people with an acquired brain injury.

- What ideas do you have about starting placement?
- What ideas do you have about a nursing home for your first placement?
- What ideas do you have about nursing individuals with an acquired brain injury?
- Can you make connections between ideas or develop some ideas further?

_____

_____

_____

_____

_____

Undertaking a free-writing exercise as above is a way of anticipatory reflection. You might have considered practical aspects such as travelling, arranging your childcare or parking. Whilst this is important for you, it is not particularly related to what or how you will learn from this experience (although thinking about this in advance might help you to become more organised). You might also have started to realise that you don't really know very much at all about acquired brain injury; so, you could set some learning goals to get a better understanding of what this means. Reading about the anatomy and physiology of, and caring for, people with an acquired brain injury and their families (e.g., Waugh and Grant [2005, p 179-181] and Holloway et al. [2019]) will help you to prepare for the nursing interventions that you will be taking part in, so this is related to what and how you will learn and will help you to maximise your learning. You might also have some concerns about how much there will be to learn in a nursing home environment. In order to learn from your experiences, it is important to remain open to the possibility that learning can take place in any and every setting where there are people requiring care, and this includes nursing homes.

So, you can see how you might start to reflect in order to learn before the nursing encounter. Try anticipatory reflection before you go into your allocated placements. You might want to start to keep a record of your thoughts and reflections so that you can come back to your ideas as you gain more nursing knowledge throughout your preregistration programme. There are some tips for creating and keeping a learning journal later in this chapter.

 TIP

For free writing for anticipatory reflection
- Start by jotting down all ideas on a particular topic on paper before undertaking any reading.
- Try not to think too much at the start; just get your ideas out. Your ideas do not need to be complete sentences with proper spelling, punctuation or grammar.
- Try and set yourself a timeframe: say 10 minutes to write everything that comes into your mind, even if it does not make sense at this stage.
- After 10 minutes, start to see if you can make connections between ideas or develop some ideas further.

Using painting to refine skills of reflection

The following is a case study of a small group exercise that you might want to try to enhance your ability to reflect. It is based on an exercise that was undertaken with a group of preregistration nursing students (McAndrew and Roberts, 2015).

CASE STUDY

Jyoti is a first-year nursing student, and she is asked to take 30 minutes to paint a picture of what she believes nursing to be. The tutors ask her to think carefully about the colours and why she chose them, as well as the images that she created.

Jyoti and each member of the group then explain the 'story' of their picture to everyone else in the group. The group is encouraged to ask questions of each other and generate discussion about what they believe nursing to be.

- You may want to undertake this exercise at the beginning of each year of your nursing programme and see whether your ideas about nursing change and, more importantly, see how your description of the picture develops over time.
- By starting to think about your ideas about nursing, together with some of the questions posed earlier in this chapter about your values and beliefs, you are starting to reflect. You are starting to think about your nurse identity and how you might practice as a nursing student and, ultimately, as a registered nurse.
- You may like to access the paper by McAndrew and Roberts (2015) (in the reference list) and see if any of your ideas are similar to those students.

Reflecting in and after action: noticing why things went well

Noticing and learning from what goes well is an important aspect of reflection. As you progress through your nurse education, you will learn to observe and notice a range of different cues from either the individual or the environment (or both) and draw these together. Being able to notice effectively will help you to focus on what needs to be done and therefore improve your practice as a future nurse.

When a nursing encounter goes well, try and think about what you noticed.

Consider the environment: Where were you in relation to the patient? Was there anything about the space that, looking back, could be considered important? Examples are room temperature, windows and light, seating arrangements and noise levels.

Nonverbal cues: Consider any facial expressions or body language that you observed and that you interpreted correctly; for example, were you able to see that a patient was in pain, even though they did not actually tell you this? What was it about the person's posture and demeanour that you could notice? Can you recall anything about your own body language that, looking back, may have been significant in helping this encounter to go well?

_____

_____

_____

_____

CASE STUDY

Stephen is a first-year mental health nursing student; he has just finished a week with a community mental health team, visiting patients in their own homes. Stephen's practice supervisor compliments Stephen on his interpersonal skills with one of the clients.

- What sort of things might Stephen think about to apply this idea of noticing when having to ask questions to assess patients in other settings?
- What cues might he look for, and how might he interpret these?
- How did he use the information gained to respond appropriately? Consider all senses.

There may be times during your preregistration nurse education where things do not go as planned, or you may feel that things did not go well. In a study of medical and nursing students' experiences of emotional challenges, Weurlander et al. (2018, p 74) highlight that 'confronting patients' illness and death, unprofessional behaviour among healthcare professionals, dilemmas regarding patient treatment, students relating to patients as individuals and not diagnoses, and using patients for their own learning' were common areas where students were emotionally challenged. The paper presents some compelling data extracts from students about these challenges. You might want to access the paper (in the reference list) and start to think about some of these emotional challenges.

GAINING CONFIDENCE

Introducing models of reflection

Several models or frameworks exist that are designed to help you to reflect in a logical sequence. The models are also designed to ensure that you consider your experience from a number of different perspectives. At this point, it's crucial to emphasise that no single model holds superiority over another in terms of ease or effectiveness. The key lies in selecting the model that best aligns with your preferences and needs. The choice of model may vary depending on the specific situation or incident or your current level of practice. The primary objective is to utilise the chosen model to learn from experience and enhance your future practice when encountering similar situations. Since reflection centres around learning from practice, it is essential to explore a range of models and identify those that resonate with you and prove helpful. Different models may offer varying levels of support in different scenarios, leading you to employ more than one model to bolster your learning process.

This section of the chapter will introduce you to two commonly used models, but there are others that may be used in practice or as part of your preregistration nurse education programme. We will provide some examples to show how the models can be used to structure your thoughts and demonstrate your learning through the experience of being a nursing student.

What? So what? Now what? Model of reflection

Rolfe et al. (2001) created a simply structured but effective model for reflection consisting of three straightforward questions: What? So what? Now what?

See Table 5.2 for how to use the Rolfe, Freshwater and Jasper model of reflection.

Example

Doran et al. (2020) use the 'What? So what? Now what? model and outline a reflection from a second-year nursing student (Doran) as she cared for a couple in a community setting. If you access and read the

---

TABLE 5.2 USING THE ROLFE, FRESHWATER AND JASPER MODEL OF REFLECTION

What?	So what?	Now what?
• Is the problem/ difficulty/reason for being stuck/reason for feeling bad/reason we don't get on? • Was my role in the situation? • Was i trying to achieve? • Actions did i take? • Was the response of others? • Were the consequences for the student? Myself? Others? • Feelings did it evoke in the student? Myself? Others? • Was good/bad about the experience?	• Does this tell me/teach me/imply/mean about me/my class/others/our relationship/my patient's care/the model of care I am using/my attitudes/ my patient's attitudes? • Was going through my mind as I acted? • Did I base my actions on? • Other knowledge can I bring to the situation? • Could/should I have done to make it better? • Is my new understanding of the situation? • Broader issues arise from the situation?	• Do I need to do in order to make things better/stop being stuck/ improve my teaching/ resolve the situation/feel better/get on better, etc.? • Broader issues need to be considered if this action is to be successful? • Might be the consequences of this action?

paper by Doran et al. (2020), which is in the reference list note how the paper is written in the first person and the model is visible.

TIP

When writing a reflective assignment, it is a good idea to use the sections of the model you have chosen as subheadings to structure it. Also, don't forget to add the model itself to your reference list!

Importantly, the student is able to consider the impact of caring for Susan and her husband:

'Before my community placement, I felt that delivering compassionate care was something I was good at, but I was not consciously aware how I was doing this or thinking about the impact I was having on my patients. Exploring the evidence that underpins compassion has taught me that nurses need to demonstrate their understanding of a patient's situation through listening, observing and respectful questioning. I have learned that it is important to see the patient (and their family members) as people first, rather than focusing on their problems. It has become important to me to work with them to find a way to resolve their issues so that their quality of life can be enhanced'.

(Doran et al., 2020, p 19).

Gibbs model of reflection

This model of reflection is perhaps the best known and one of the most widely used by nursing students when writing reflective assignments. Gibbs (1988)'s reflective cycle is a framework for examining experiences and, given its cyclic nature, lends itself particularly well to repeated experiences, allowing you to learn and plan from things that either went well or didn't go well. The model has six linked elements that are usually depicted as a cycle or circle. See Fig. 5.3.

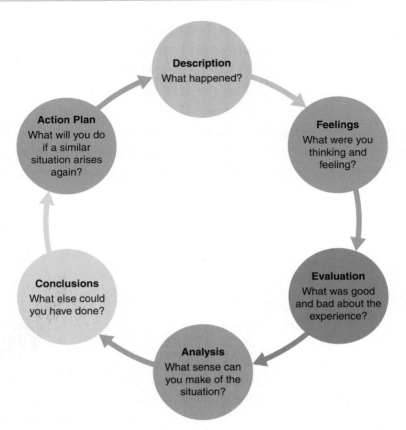

Fig. 5.3   Gibbs reflective cycle.

Gibbs (1988)'s model provides a logical structure for students to gain meaningful understanding from their experiences. It is straightforward and uncomplicated, making it ideal to use when you are starting out with learning to reflect on your practice (Duffy, 2007). The focus should be on you and your experiences; each element of the model carries equal importance.

You can work through the model by talking to your practice supervisor or one of your peers, or you can use the model to structure a reflective assignment—more about that later! Here are some example key questions that you might ask yourself which relate to each stage:

- **Description:** Start here. Only state the facts of the situation: where the event took place, who was there and what your role in the situation was. Try to avoid including aspects of how you felt at this stage. Focus on the event itself. Write as concisely as possible, avoiding assumptions and sweeping statements.

- **Feelings:** This section can be tricky, particularly if the event did not go as planned or if you found the event emotionally difficult, but it is important to consider your emotions, how you felt before, during and after the event. Were there particular things that happened or things that were said that influenced how you felt? Remember that feelings do not have to be negative: you can focus on events that went well and explore why that was the case.

- **Evaluation:** Here, it is important to think about whether the event went well or not so well, but this should be balanced, and consider the totality of the situation with all its relevant parts. If you are writing a reflective assignment, you should introduce some literature to support your ideas about whether the situation went well or not.

- **Analysis:** This involves a closer look at each element of what took place: what did you or others do well in this situation, why didn't things turn out the way you had expected and what was your part in this? It is important to identify gaps in knowledge, skills or experiences that need to be filled.

- **Conclusions:** Provide some insight into your own actions and behaviour. What else could you have done? What other approaches are you aware of that could have been used?

- **Action plan:** Plan ahead so that you will feel better prepared for similar situations. What elements of your practice will you repeat, and which will you change? What is the evidence base for your decisions? Note how the action plan takes you back to description: reminding you to reflect on similar experiences and continually grow as a learner and future nurse.

Examples

Mlinar Reljić et al. (2019) describe research that explores a group of Slovenian nursing students' experiences of their first placement. The students kept reflective diaries to facilitate their reflection. Reflection enabled the students to express their emotions and feelings; the authors suggest that this leads to better insight.

Similarly, O'Regan and Fawcett (2006) provide an example of the Gibbs model being used to structure reflection following the bathing of a patient by a nursing student. Each section of the model is visible and attended to in turn. This paper was written in 2006; remember, nursing knowledge is constantly being updated, so there will always be new evidence that you will need to consider and then make a judgement about whether to apply that new evidence to the care of patients.

Reading critically

This section of the chapter provides some advice about reading and writing using critical thinking skills. According to Ross (2020, p 62), 'the key to critical thinking and writing is critical reading'. Reading critically, like many other things during your nursing education, is a skill that can be practised and learned. Suggested key aspects of learning to read critically are:

- Focus intensely and engage with the text.
- Access the level of literature that suits you, remembering to build on this as your confidence develops.
- Make your environment one that is conducive to thinking e.g., quiet, no interruptions.
- Study at a time that suits your needs.
- Focus on the author's message and identify the key points: separate what is relevant from what is not. Do this by reading the whole text first to get a flavour of the work and then select one paragraph at a time for closer scrutiny. Consciously ask: 'What is this author telling me?'
- Be sceptical or open-minded.

Ross (2020) offers valuable tips for becoming a better critical reader and more sceptical. As you progress through your nursing education, you will be expected to read and engage with nursing research. There are several frameworks that you can use to help you become more critical in your reading of different types of research (see Chapter 8). Rees (2010, p 178-179) provides two frameworks to facilitate critique of qualitative and quantitative research. He outlines a series of questions that the reader should be asking of the literature. He points out that, initially, when using the framework, it will take you longer to read a research article but that, actually, this is helpful, as you will learn to see things that you might otherwise miss. With confidence, speed increases, and the language associated with complex critiquing skills develops.

Writing it down

Keeping a reflective journal

Being able to demonstrate critical thinking in your academic work is likely to be a part of your nurse education programme. Here, we offer some advice for keeping a reflective journal and outline some skills for writing reflective assignments and demonstrating critical thinking in academic work.

A learning journal can be used as a private space where you 'sit' with your thoughts and experiences, make connections and, ultimately, take an active role in your learning—this is true for both nursing students and registered nurses. It is a good idea to keep a learning or reflective journal. You can decide whether you keep this as a private learning tool or whether you show it to your practice supervisor or personal tutor. See the following quote from a nursing student who kept a reflective journal during the pandemic.

'Since the beginning of my nurse training, I have kept a reflective journal. There is something rather cathartic about seeing, concretised on the page before me, thoughts and feelings that were, until that point in time, abstract, intangible emotions. Night after night, I would return home from placement and write. Some evenings I would write for hours in an almost desperate attempt to make sense of what I had witnessed, or what I had learned. In many respects, my journal became my therapist, my confidante, my non-judgemental sounding board of how I was coping.

In readiness for this final reflection, I re-read my COVID entries. It was intriguing to note that a greater portion of them contemplate

Continued

> *the human condition in the face of a pandemic—the thoughts, fears, hopes and sometimes despair of my patients and their relatives. My entries taught me about not just the ability to survive a clinical placement in a pandemic, but also how to survive, more profoundly, as a human being'.*
>
> **(Townsend, 2020, p 973)**

Reflective assignments

As part of your preregistration programme, you may be required to submit reflective assignments or illustrate your work with examples drawn from clinical practice. Reflective writing is where you are expected to demonstrate what you have learned from a nursing or patient care encounter. Since the account is about you and what you have learned, you should be visible in the assignment, so, unlike other types of academic writing, you can write in the first person.

 TIP

- Maintain anonymity and confidentiality when writing reflective accounts (see Chapter 10). Never use a person's real name; use a pseudonym (made-up name), and the placement or location of the ward or service should also remain anonymous. So, for example, you might write: *'I first met Mr Patel (a pseudonym) as a first-year nursing student when I was allocated to a diabetic outpatient clinic in a local NHS Trust. My practice supervisor, Staff Nurse Smith (a pseudonym), introduced me to Mr Patel, who was attending clinic for follow-up, having recently been diagnosed with type 2 diabetes'.*
- It is important to write about something that you were party to as a nursing student. Don't be tempted to make a story up; this defeats the objective of the entire exercise. You should demonstrate your learning through your experience. It is more important that you learn from the experience rather than being able to score

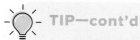

TIP—cont'd

good marks and learn very little. So, be warned! The situation that you write about should be real.

- It is important that you show that you are continuously questioning your personal assumptions, values and beliefs, the nursing profession and the world in which we live.
- There is no substitute for wide reading around the subject area. You need to allow sufficient time to read and think about how this knowledge contributes to your learning. Narrow reading will be evident in your work and will be reflected in the grade you achieve.

TRANSFERRING LEARNING AND CRITICAL THINKING TO PRACTICE

Throughout your journey as a nursing student, you will be encouraged to develop the use of critical thinking skills and utilise these within everyday practice. The need for critical thinking in nursing has been accentuated in response to the rapidly changing healthcare environment. As long ago as 1997, Oermann suggested that critical thinking is not developed through one lecture or one clinical experience; instead, skills in thinking develop over time through varied experiences, and this remains true. Nurses must think critically to provide effective care while coping with the expansion in role associated with the complexities of current healthcare systems.

Beginning to use critical thinking and reflection as a nursing student

So, what is critical thinking, and how do you start to apply critical thinking into practice?

Here are some definitions to consider in the understanding and application of critical thinking:

Alfaro-Lefevre (2019) suggests that critical thinking is a complex, dynamic process formed by attitudes and strategic skills, with the aim of achieving a specific goal or objective. The attitudes, including the critical-thinking attitudes, constitute an important part of the idea of good care of the good professional.

Critical thinking is characterised as being:

- Organised
- Structured
- Specific
- Inquisitive about the intentions, facts and reasons behind an idea or action
- Involves formulating questions to gain a deeper understanding of what is happening and why (Alfaro-Lefevre, 2019)

Interestingly, knowledge is necessary but, on its own, is not enough for healthcare workers to provide the appropriate healthcare services; the ability to think about and effectively use knowledge is also an essential element (Lunney, 2009)—in other words, critical thinking. It is important to know where and when to apply such knowledge and to which people in your care. Similarly, Papathanasiou et al. (2014) define critical thinking as the mental process of active and skilful perception, analysis, synthesis and evaluation of collected information through observation, experience and communication, leading to a decision for action.

 TIP

- **Critical thinking is a process that everyone has the capacity to master, including you! But your journey to being a future nurse takes time, and once registered as a nurse, your learning and growth will continue throughout your career.**
- **The first vital step would be to learn from practice supervisors and practice assessors with strong practice experience when you access placements in health and social care settings.**
- **Whilst on your placement, consider asking a range of registered professionals how they apply learning and critical thinking into practice. Ask them to talk through their thought processes when undertaking a complex task.**

Fleming (2020) states the concept of critical thinking has been defined in many complex ways, but for students new to the concept, it can best be summed up as thinking and judging for yourself. When you develop critical thinking skills, you will learn to evaluate information that you hear and process information that you collect while recognising your implicit biases. You will analyse the evidence that is presented to you to make sure it is sound. Critical thinking involves suspending your beliefs to explore and question topics from a 'blank page' point of view. It also involves the ability to distinguish fact from opinion when exploring a topic.

Have a look at this case study designed to help develop critical thinking skills.

CASE STUDY

A group of first-year nursing students have been assigned the task of conducting a tour for aliens who are visiting the earth and observing human life. The group is asked to imagine riding along in a blimp, viewing the landscape below. The group floats over a professional football stadium. How would you explain what's going on to the alien group?

The aliens ask several important questions:

- What is a game?
- Why are there no female players?
- Why do people get so excited about watching other people play games?
- What is a team?
- Why can't the people in the seats go down on the field and join in?

So, by now, you should be starting to realise that when we try and answer these questions, we carry around certain assumptions and values. We support a certain team, for instance, because it makes us feel like we're a part of a community. This sense of community is a value that matters to some people more than others. Furthermore, when trying to explain team sports to an alien, you must explain the value we place on winning and losing. When you think like an alien tour guide, you are forced to take a deeper look at our actions and values. Sometimes they don't sound logical from the outside looking in.

Do you think you know the difference between fact and opinion? It's not always easy to discern. When you visit websites, do you believe everything you read? The abundance of available information makes it more important than ever for students to develop critical thinking skills.

If you don't learn the difference between fact and opinion, you may end up reading and watching things that continue to reinforce beliefs and assumptions you already own.

 Read each statement below. Do you think these are facts or opinions? This can be completed alone or with a peer.

- My mum is the best mum on earth.
- My dad is taller than your dad.
- My telephone number is difficult to memorise.
- The deepest part of the ocean is 35,813 feet deep.
- Dogs make better pets than turtles.
- Smoking is bad for your health.
- Eighty-five percent of all cases of lung cancer in the United States are caused by smoking.
- If you flatten and stretch out a Slinky toy, it will be 87 feet long.
- Slinky toys are fun.
- One out of every 100 American citizens is colour blind.
- Two out of 10 UK citizens are boring.

_____

_____

_____

_____

You probably found some of the statements easy to judge but others difficult. If you can effectively debate the truthfulness of a statement with other members of your nursing cohort, then it's most likely an opinion.

TIP

Here are some simple steps on starting to get you thinking critically as a nursing student:

- Identify a problem or issue.
- Create inferences on why the problem exists and how it can be solved.
- Collect information or data on the issue through research.
- Organise and sort data and findings.
- Develop and execute solutions.
- Analyse which solutions worked or didn't work.
- Identify ways to improve the solution.

Critical thinking is a specific way of using your mind. It's your ability to objectively judge information rather than believing everything you are told. Critical thinking is something you'll do every day as a nurse, and honestly, you probably do it in your regular non-nurse life as well. It's basically stopping, looking at a situation, identifying a solution and trying it out. Critical thinking in nursing is just that but in a clinical setting.

CONCLUSION

Reflection and critical thinking are key mechanisms by which you will learn from your experience. According to some authors, they are key to becoming an expert practitioner (Benner, 1984). Critical thinking supports reflection, organising thoughts, identifying strengths and areas for improvement and integrating the evidence base to ensure ethically sound optimal person-centred decisions.

This chapter has outlined three types of reflection: anticipatory, reflection in action and reflection on action. All three are important skills in your journey towards being a future nurse. Reflection starts with and is all about you and your practice, so it is important to have insight and understanding of yourself and your beliefs about health, illness and nursing. We have offered some top tips, case studies and opportunities for you to consider and make your own notes to help you to get started with reflection and critical thinking. You might try to use the two models that we have described too.

Gradually, as you start to use reflection and critical thinking to help you to make sense of, find meaning in and learn from practice, you will be able to draw conclusions about the nursing interventions you have used and transfer your learning to a similar situation or to other nursing contexts. In doing this, you will assemble a personal library of experience that you can draw on to keep learning throughout your nursing career.

Now you have finished this chapter. Please make notes on what you have learned.

_____

_____

_____

_____

_____

_____

_____

_____

_____

_____

_____

_____

_____

_____

_____

_____

_____

_____

_____

_____

_____

_____

REFERENCES

Alfaro-Lefevre, R. (2019) *Critical Thinking, Clinical Reasoning and Clinical Judgment. A Practical Approach*, 7th ed. Edinburgh: Elsevier.

Benner. P. (1984) *From Novice to Expert: Excellence and Power in Clinical Nursing Practice*. New York: Addison-Wesley Publishing Co.

Doran, D., Phillips, J. and Board, M. (2020) 'Compassionate care in the community: reflections of a student nurse', *British Journal of Community Nursing*, 25(1), pp. 16–21. Available at: https://doi.org/10.12968/bjcn.2020.25.1.16.

Duffy, A. (2007) 'A concept analysis of reflective practice: determining its value to nurses', *British Journal of Nursing*, 16(22), pp. 1400–1407. Available at: https://doi.org/10.12968/bjon.2007.16.22.27771.

Flemming, G. (2020) *Introduction to critical thinking*. Available at: https://www.thoughtco.com/introduction-to-critical-thinking-1857079 (Accessed 29.1.24)

Gibbs, G. (1988) *Learning by Doing: A Guide to a Teaching And Learning Methods*. Oxford: Further Educational Unit - Polytechnic.

Holloway, M., Orr, D., and Clark-Wilson, J. (2019) 'Experiences of challenges and support among family members of people with acquired brain injury: a qualitative study in the UK', *Brain Injury,* 33(4), pp. 401–411, DOI: 10.1080/02699052.2019.1566967

Howatson-Jones, L. (2010) *Reflective Practice in Nursing.* (Transforming Nursing Practice Series). Poole: Learning Matters.

Jasper, M. (2013) *Beginning Reflective Practice,* 2nd ed. Andover: Cengage Learning

Lucy, D. (2012) 'Prisoner's story inspired me to explore my prejudiced attitudes'. *Nursing Standard.* 26(43). p. 29.

Lunney, M. (ed.) (2009) *Critical Thinking To Achieve Positive Health Outcomes: Nursing Case Studies and Analyses*, 2nd ed. Kaukauna: NANDA International Wiley-Blackwell.

McAndrew, S. and Roberts, D. (2015) 'Reflection in nurse education: promoting deeper thinking through the use of painting', *Reflective Practice*, 16(2), pp. 206–217. Available at: https://doi.org/10.1080/14623943.2014.992406.

Mlinar Reljić, N., Pajnkihar, M. and Fekonja, Z. (2019) 'Self-reflection during first clinical practice: the experiences of nursing students', *Nurse Education Today*, 72, pp. 61–66. Available at: https://doi.org/10.1016/j.nedt.2018.10.019.

Murdoch-Eaton, D. and Sandars, J. (2014) 'Reflection: moving from a mandatory ritual to meaningful professional development', *Archives of Disease in Childhood*, 99(3), pp. 279–283. Available at: https://doi.org/10.1136/archdischild-2013-303948.

Nicol, J. S. and Dosser, I. (2016) 'Understanding reflective practice', *Nursing Standard,* 30(36), pp. 34–40.

Nursing and Midwifery Council (2018a) *Future nurse: Standards of proficiency for registered nurse*. London: Nursing and Midwifery Council. Available at: https://www.nmc.org.uk/globalassets/sitedocuments/education-standards/future-nurse-proficiencies.pdf (Accessed: 21 August 2022).

Nursing and Midwifery Council (2018b) *The code. Professional standards of practice and behaviour for nurses, midwives and nursing associates*. London: Nursing and Midwifery Council. Available at: https://www.nmc.org.uk/globalassets/sitedocuments/nmc-publications/nmc-code.pdf (Accessed: 13 November 2022). –28. Available at: https://doi.org/10.1097/00006223-199709000-00011.

O' Regan, H. and Fawcett, T. (2006) 'Learning to nurse: reflections on bathing a patient'. *Nursing Standard,* 20(46), pp. 60–64. doi: 10.1097/00006223-199709000-00011.

Oermann, M. H. (1997) 'Evaluating critical thinking in clinical practice'. *Nurse educator*, 22(5), 25–28. https://doi.org/10.1097/00006223-199709000-00011

Papathanasiou, I., Kleisiaris, C., Fradelos, E., Kakou, K. and Kourkouta, L. (2014) 'Critical thinking: the development of an essential skill for nursing students'. *Acta Informatica Medica*, 22(4), p. 283–286. Available at: https://doi.org/10.5455/aim.2014.22.

Price, B. and Harrington, A. (2010) *Critical Thinking and Writing for Nursing Students. (Transforming Nursing Practice Series)*. Poole: Learning Matters.

Rees, C. (2010). 'Evaluating and appraising evidence to underpin nursing practice'. In Holland, K. and Rees, C. (Eds). *Nursing: Evidence-Based Practice Skills*. Oxford: Oxford University Press.

Rolfe, G., Freshwater, D., and Jasper, M. (2001) *Critical reflection in nursing and the helping professions: A user's guide*. Basingstoke: Palgrave Macmillan.

Rolfe, G., Jasper, M. and Freshwater, D. (2010) *Critical Reflection in Practice*, 2nd ed. Basingstoke: Palgrave Macmillan.

Ross, T. (2020) 'Skills for critical thinking'. In Ghisoni, M. and Murphy, P. (Eds) *Study Skills for Nursing, Health and Social Care*. Oxford: Lantern Publishing.

Schon, D. A. (1983) *The Reflective Practitioner*. London: Temple Smith.

Schon, D. A. (1987) *Educating the Reflective Practitioner: How Professionals Think in Action*. San Francisco: Jossey-Bass.

Townsend, M. J. (2020) 'Learning to nurse during the pandemic: a student's reflections'. *British journal of nursing*, 29(16), 972–973. https://doi.org/10.12968/bjon.2020.29.16.972

Van Manen, M. (1991) *The Tact of Teaching*. New York: State University of New York Press.

Waugh, A. and Grant, A. (2005) *Ross and Wilson: Anatomy and Physiology in Health and Illness (9th edition)*. 11th edn. Edinburgh: Churchill Livingstone. Available at: https://napier-repository.worktribe.com/output/256702/ross-and-wilson-anatomy-and-physiology-in-health-and-illness-9th-edition (Accessed: 22 July 2023).

Weurlander, M., Lönn, A., Seeberger, A., Broberger, E., Hult, H. and Wernerson, A. (2018) 'How do medical and nursing students experience emotional challenges during clinical placements?', *International Journal of Medical Education*, 9, pp. 74–82. Available at: https://doi.org/10.5116/ijme.5a88.1f80.

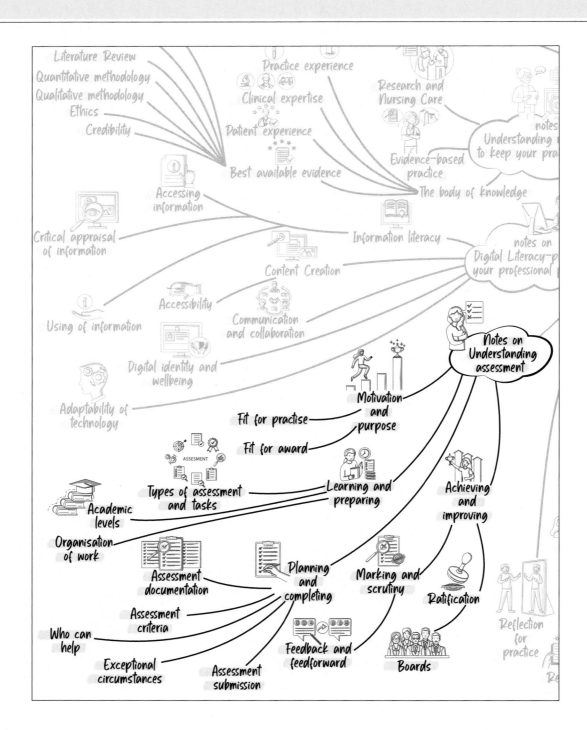

NOTES ON UNDERSTANDING ASSESSMENT

Melanie Hayward (she/her)

INTRODUCTION

This chapter explores the concept of assessment in preregistration nursing education. It will help you understand the importance of developing motivation and purpose for assessment, as well as the significance of understanding assessment tasks. You will learn what is expected of you in these tasks and how to best prepare for success. Additionally, you will be able to identify the various resources available to support you in planning, completing and submitting assessment tasks, including associated documentation. This chapter will also guide you on how to evaluate your performance and what steps to take if things do not go as expected. Furthermore, it will support you in exploring strategies to improve for future assessments and the invaluable assistance provided by supervisors, assessors and academics, ensuring continuous growth and development throughout your nursing education. By the end of this chapter, you will have a solid foundation for understanding assessments for nursing students and be equipped with the knowledge, skills and resources necessary to approach them with confidence.

THE LEARNER JOURNEY

Most people do not like being assessed. It feels as if you are being judged, and there is always a risk of failure. Students can feel stupid if they make a mistake or do not achieve a certain grade; this can cause feelings of inadequacy and lower motivation (Kivunja, 2015). However, assessment is not about critiquing performance, it is about facilitating meaningful active learning (Culha, 2019). Your tutors, lecturers, academics and practice assessors are all on your side; they want you to succeed and will help you do so.

> To begin with, take some time to consider an answer to the following question, 'Why do nursing students undertake assessments?'
>
> _____
>
> _____
>
> _____
>
> _____

Assessment is a central activity within any learning process in formal education. It allows students to demonstrate what knowledge they have gained, skills they have learned and behaviours they have developed. The feedback and feedforward received by students following the completion of any assessment are aimed at supporting reflection on current achievement and providing information and guidance on how to improve.

Preregistration nursing assessment ensures students are fit for practice and their degree award. By this, we mean guaranteeing students' understanding, abilities and attitude to meet both professional and academic expectations. The Nursing and Midwifery Council (NMC) (2018a, 2018b, 2018c, 2018d, 2018e) sets the registerable standard you must meet and uphold, and the proficiencies you must be competent in, to ensure high-quality, evidence-based, safe and compassionate person-centred care. They also outline the expectations of approved nursing programmes for universities and practice learning or employer partners (placement areas) to follow. The Quality Assurance Agency (2014, 2018a) and Scottish Credit and Qualifications Framework (SCQF) (2022) outline key principles of effective assessment and the required academic level for each year.

MOTIVATION FOR AND PURPOSE OF ASSESSMENT

CASE STUDY

Ben, a first-year adult nursing student, started his degree just over 2 months ago and is already feeling the pressure. He enjoyed his first 6 weeks of lectures at university and was excited to start his current placement, but the 12-hour shifts and 1.5-hour travelling time each way is starting to take its toll. His partner is supportive, but organising childcare and studying at home are difficult. He is starting to worry that he is not being the best partner or father and can't stop thinking about the fact that when he qualifies, he will earn less than the job he left behind.

Many students study nursing for similar reasons, perhaps a personal experience of healthcare or caring, a passion to help others, a desire to work as part of a skilled team or maybe wanting to join the most trusted profession (Ipsos, 2022). You will have specific and individual reasons.

What are your reasons for studying nursing?

_____

_____

_____

_____

SOCIAL MEDIA

@crazygirlfriend

'My main goal in life is to change people's lives and that's why I decided to study nursing. The feeling that it gives me to know that I made someone's day or that I saved a life brings me so much happiness and motivates me every day'.

As highlighted in the case study and Chapter 1, remaining motivated throughout your studies can be challenging due to various factors such as life priorities, financial pressures, commuting and long hours of learning both at university and placement (Mills et al., 2020). But it can be especially tough if you also find studying difficult or assessment anxiety provoking. A key way to keep motivated is to remind yourself of your 'why'. No matter how determined you are to be a nurse or how dedicated you are to your studies, you will struggle to be successful unless you 'learn how to learn' (Chapter 2), develop key study skills (Chapter 3) and understand what you are expected to learn and how you are required to demonstrate this learning (Chapters 4 and 5).

Assessment is intended to drive learning behaviour; therefore, well-designed assessment is crucial for effective learning (Scott, 2020). You may hear your lecturers, or notice your programme documentation, referring to a strategy for teaching, learning and assessment. This is the approach used to develop, deliver and evaluate an effective teaching and learning experience for students.

NMC | THE NMC SAYS

5.1 'Curricula and assessments are designed, developed, delivered and evaluated to ensure that students achieve the proficiencies and outcomes for their approved programme'.

Your university will have an evidence-based policy which outlines their vision for high-quality, purposeful education. This, in addition to the higher education standards set out by the Quality Assurance Agency (2018b) and the professional standards of education and training set out by the NMC (2018a, 2018b, 2018c), will have informed your nursing programme's teaching, learning and assessment strategy. All assessment within your course, whether academic or practice based, has been carefully planned and designed as part of this strategy to support your academic progress as well as prepare you for the real world of qualified nursing practice.

Fit for practice

For UK nursing students, being fit to practise at qualification and therefore able to register with the NMC means having been successfully assessed to have the professional knowledge, skills and behaviours expected of all registered nurses. It requires having the ability, as well as good health and character, to safely, compassionately and effectively, across all care settings, nurse individuals and families of all ages and developmental stages with varying health needs. Professional expectations are set out in the code (NMC, 2018e) and professional competencies in the standards of proficiency for registered nurses (NMC, 2018d).

Fit for award

Nursing students in the United Kingdom have to successfully complete a minimum of an undergraduate first-degree qualification (NMC, 2018a). In England, Wales and Northern Ireland, the required standard, or difficulty level, of academic work is set by the Frameworks for Higher Education Qualification (FHEQ) descriptors (Quality Assurance Agency, 2014) and, in Scotland, the SCQF (2022). Each year or part of study is aligned to an FHEQ or SCQF level which needs to be attained through passing corresponding levelled assessments to progress to the next and finally qualify. In England, individuals studying at the undergraduate level can study a self-funded or an employer-funded apprenticeship programme. A registered nurse degree apprenticeship (RNDA) can be undertaken by individuals who meet the entry requirement and are employed by eligible NHS or other healthcare providers (Department of Health and Social Care, 2016). If you are an apprentice, your programme will have also been written against the RNDA occupational standard (Institute for Apprenticeships and Technical Education, 2022), which defines the occupational nurse profile, a list of duties, as well as the knowledge, skills and behaviours aligned with the NMC (2018e, 2018d) proficiencies and code. See the diagram as follows, which outlines the UK higher education context of how qualification types are arranged relative to each other and the academic levels students have to progress through at each stage or year of their programme (Fig. 6.1).

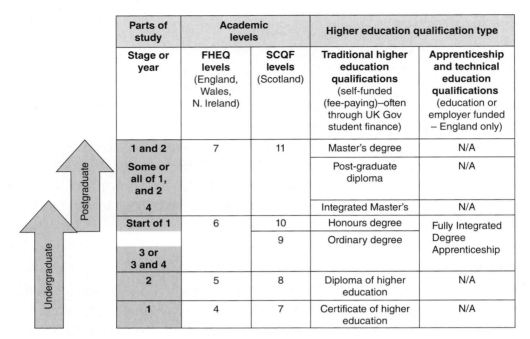

Parts of study	Academic levels		Higher education qualification type	
Stage or year	FHEQ levels (England, Wales, N. Ireland)	SCQF levels (Scotland)	Traditional higher education qualifications (self-funded (fee-paying)–often through UK Gov student finance)	Apprenticeship and technical education qualifications (education or employer funded – England only)
1 and 2	7	11	Master's degree	N/A
Some or all of 1, and 2			Post-graduate diploma	N/A
4			Integrated Master's	N/A
Start of 1	6	10	Honours degree	Fully Integrated Degree Apprenticeship
3 or 3 and 4		9	Ordinary degree	
2	5	8	Diploma of higher education	N/A
1	4	7	Certificate of higher education	N/A

Fig. 6.1 UK higher education context of qualification types. *FHEQ,* Frameworks for Higher Education Qualification; *SCQF,* Scottish Credit and Qualifications Framework.

Practice focus

In practice, you are assessed against professional values, clinical proficiencies (NMC, 2018d) and specific learning outcomes or objectives relevant to your placement areas that have been agreed upon with your practice assessor. These are outlined and documented in your practice assessment document (PAD). This may be a paper document or an electronic document known as the ePAD. The expected level of your understanding, its application to practice and subsequent degree of skill competence are only broadly aligned with the FHEQ or SCQF levels, reflecting the dynamic nature, unique demands and complexity of practice. Clinical skills and caring experiences do not fully align, placements are diverse, health and social care environments are unpredictable and learning and assessment processes and support differ as you access various practice environments and practice supervisors and assessors change.

How does it fit together?

Nursing academics at your university have designed your programme focused on the expected standards applied to your chosen field(s)—adult, child, learning disability and/or mental health—of practice using constructive alignment (Biggs, 1996) like this:

- **Programme**: Each consists of a curriculum with overarching **course-level learning outcomes** or **objectives**, made up of multiple modules or units of study, completed over 2–5 years, depending on whether it is:
  - Part-time or full-time
  - Fee paying or apprenticeship
  - Undergraduate ordinary, honours or integrated master's degree or a postgraduate diploma or master's degree
  - Single field of practice or dual field of practice qualification.
- Each **module or unit** has its own
  - **Learning outcomes** or **objectives**, mapped to the NMC (2018d) standards of proficiency for registered nurses, aligned to the relevant FHEQ or SCQF academic level
  - **Teaching and learning activities** designed to enable you to meet those learning outcomes or objectives
  - **Assessments,** one or more formative and summative. Depending on how many there are, they will be linked to some or all of the learning outcomes or objectives to enable you to demonstrate that you have met them.

NMC

THE NMC SAYS

5.11 'Assessment is mapped to the curriculum and occurs throughout the programme to determine student progression'.

See the following for a pictorial representation of an example of constructive alignment at undergraduate level for an ordinary degree in Scotland or honours degree in England, Wales or Northern Ireland (Fig. 6.2).

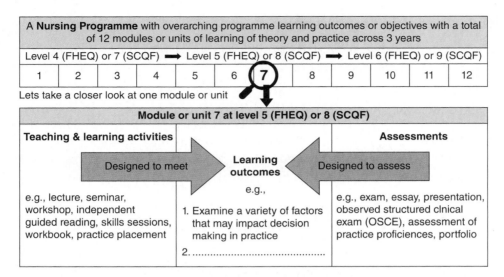

Fig. 6.2   Representation of an example of constructive alignment. *FHEQ,* Frameworks for Higher Education Qualification; *SCQF,* Scottish Credit and Qualifications Framework.

LEARNING ABOUT AND PREPARING FOR ASSESSMENT TASKS

Having discovered the intention of assessment in nursing programmes and how it is designed and created, we will now explore in closer detail the characteristics, types and broad expectations of assessments in both theory and practice and start to think about getting organised.

CASE STUDY

Sumaya, a first-year mental health registered nurse degree apprentice, was enthusiastic about starting her course 4 months ago and quickly got stuck in with in-person and online learning activities. She avoided looking at assessments in-depth until recently, as she felt she did not know enough to prepare for them. With less than 2 weeks left of placement and 2 weeks before her first numeracy exam and essay are due, she is beginning to panic and is worried her best won't be good enough.

It is easy to become overwhelmed by the assessment elements of your nursing programme. You may be uncertain as to exactly what you need to do, confused as to when you need to do it by or worried about failing. Anxiety about the unknown or doubt about your performance may lead to procrastination (Chapter 2). Avoiding last-minute exam revision or assignment writing and inadequate practice assessment preparation are important to avoid further stress and possible underperformance. Whatever is leading you to panic, the best way to combat negative feelings is to identify what you are finding challenging, ask yourself and others what you can do to overcome the difficulty (Chapter 1) and then engage in actions to combat them.

One of the most important things you can do to reduce assessment-related anxiety or uncertainty is to access and read the key documents and sections of your virtual learning environment (e.g., Blackboard, Moodle), which outline the upcoming expectations. Chapter 1 introduced you to these.

Formative, summative, authentic and inclusive assessment

Most theory and practice modules or units of learning will have formative and summative assessments, which should be authentic and inclusive by design. When reading through your handbooks or schemes, these aspects may not be obvious to you or named as such, but they are important for you to know to provide understanding, value and purpose when planning your studies and preparing for assessments.

NMC

THE NMC SAYS

5.8 'Assessment is fair, reliable and valid to enable students to demonstrate they have achieved the proficiencies for their programme'

Formative assessments are optional and provide feedback on what you have done well and not so well, in addition to feedforward, on how to make improvements, from your tutors, lecturers or practice assessors to enable you to be successful in your summative assessments (Duers and Brown, 2009; Koh, 2010). (See the 'Scrutiny of assessment' section.)

TABLE 6.1 FORMATIVE AND SUMMATIVE ASSESSMENT

Formative assessments	Summative assessments
• Informal activities	• Formal activities
• Embedded throughout your theoretical or practice module or unit of learning	• Normally occurs towards the end of your theoretical or practice module or unit of learning
• Supports tutors, lecturers or practice assessors to identify gaps in learning and support progression against expected learning outcomes or objectives	• Supports your tutors, lecturers or practice assessors to evaluate your performance against the expected learning outcomes or objectives
• Assists you to practice, improve your learning, prepare and complete summative assessments	• Enables you to demonstrate you have met the learning outcomes or objectives
• Optional	• Compulsory
• Both provide feedback and feedforward to support you to improve to be successful in current or future summative assessment	

Summative assessments are compulsory, formally evaluating the module or unit learning outcomes or objectives, and must be passed in order to progress through the programme. Simply put, formative assessment is assessment for learning, and summative assessment is assessment of learning. See Table 6.1, which outlines the key features and differences.

SOCIAL MEDIA
@reboverend_RNc

'Feedforward: enable the learner to stretch into new learning – helps them to find goal. Feedback: learning conversation. What went well, how did it feel, why and what actions could change that? Making time to do it at the time also important'.

You may have recognised, whether formative or summative, that assessment tasks differ throughout your programme. You may prefer a certain type, for example, essays rather than exams or posters rather than oral presentations. Or, like many nursing students, you may have a preference for practice assessment in placement rather than academic assessment of theoretical learning (Hunt et al., 2012). But, in order to allow students to successfully learn and then demonstrate 'what they understand or what they can do', assessments need to be authentic. Authentic assessment in a nursing programme means it effectively measures the intended learning outcomes or objectives as well as prepares students for 'real-life' nursing (Poindexter et al., 2015). This means assessments have true benefit for professional registered qualified practice (for further information, see the 'Types of assessment tasks' section).

Finally, an effective assessment should be inclusive. If you have health issues, a disability or a learning difficulty, ensure that you inform your personal tutor at the start of your studies and access the appropriate team at your university to ensure any reasonable adjustments you need are put in place (Chapter 11).

Inclusive assessment, though, is not just about meeting the additional needs of students under the Equality Act 2010. It is a good-quality non-discriminatory academic practice and should exist to enable all students to have an equal opportunity to be successful (Nieminen, 2022). It should be embedded for all learners, as not only academic and practical abilities differ but also preferred learning styles, culture, first language, prior learning experience and personal and professional circumstances. Primarily, you will observe this in two ways:

1. **Easily accessible and understood information**, e.g., logically ordered and simply worded documents, videos or voiceover presentations alongside written information explaining the assessment task
2. **Choice**, this may be *of assessment task*, e.g., an extended literature review or work-based project, or *within the assessment task*, e.g., a presentation that can be delivered in-person, online or recorded, or a clinical skill assessed through patient-facing or simulated practice. Making the right choice is important, as this can greatly affect your experience and performance.

Types of assessment tasks

You will now appreciate that there are different types of formative and summative assessment tasks, and some are more likely to be found in nursing programmes than others (Chapter 4). All assessment, like learning, is weighted equally across theory and practice. In addition, for pre-registration nursing, the NMC (2018a, 2018c) mandates the following assessment requirements:

- A health **numeracy assessment** related to nursing proficiencies and calculation of medicines to be passed at 100%
- Practice assessment facilitated and evidenced by **observations**
- Students' **self-reflections**
- The contribution of a range of people, including **service users**

Here are the most common types of theoretical and practice assessment tasks in nursing programmes.

Type of assessment task	Key features and purpose for professional practice
Case study	**What** A piece of writing analysing an organisational, professional, team or patient problem or incident. The case study may be provided, or it may be chosen by you based on your experience. This may be a piece of coursework, such as an essay or report, or may form part or the whole of a long question exam. **Why** Allows you to apply theory to practice issues to understand why things occur the way they do and use the evidence base to provide explanation and make recommendations.
Essay	**What** Persuasive writing on a particular topic or in response to a question. Has an introduction, main body and conclusion. Typically written in the third person and past tense. **Why** Allows you to demonstrate your knowledge and increased levels of analytical and critical thinking as you progress through the course. **Formative**—short essays, essay plans or introductions **Summative**—full essay expectations with a specific word count

Type of assessment task	Key features and purpose for professional practice

Examination
- **Written**

What

A set of multiple-choice, short- or long-answer questions to be completed within a specific time frame.

Why

Unseen exams are used to support you to recall information. An **open-book exam**, which allows you to refer to course materials during the exam, and a **seen exam,** where the questions are given out beforehand, test your ability to apply learning to new situations.

Formative—classroom, paper-based or interactive quizzes or practice exam questions

Summative—online or in a classroom and involves invigilation

Examples:

- Numeracy assessment consisting of drug calculations using set scenarios or a prescription/drug chart
- Using the nursing process and care planning for a patient with a certain condition based on a case study

Literature review

What

A written comprehensive analysis and critique of published evidence. Often used as the dissertation or forms part of the final academic project of the programme.

Why

Allows you to focus on and deepen your understanding of an area of nursing which is of real interest to you and to demonstrate your research knowledge.

OSCE
- **Practical**

What

A planned and coordinated examination in a simulated environment. May be used for academic and/or practice assessment. There may be one or a series of stations that mimic real-life practice scenarios where you are required to exhibit professional behaviours and/or clinical skills and associated evidence-based knowledge using a person-centred approach.

Continued

Type of assessment task	Key features and purpose for professional practice
	Why Allows you to demonstrate professional behaviours and NMC proficiencies which are difficult to assess through direct patient care, written examination or coursework. **Examples:** • Safely administer intravenous antibiotics • Undertake urinary catheterisation of a female adult patient
Observations	**What** A set of observational assessments with related feedback that take place in the practice environment. Some may require a written description, evaluation or reflection and/or receiving written feedback from service users and professionals. Areas of observation include professional values, clinical proficiencies, episodes of care and medicine management. **Why** Allows you to demonstrate understanding of and ability to practice as per the NMC code and your competency across the NMC proficiencies. Require a greater depth of knowledge as you progress and additional more advanced skills to meet the specific care needs of people in your chosen field(s) of nursing practice.
Portfolio • **Paper based** • **Online** (e-portfolio)	**What** An individual professional record of your learning, reflections and achievements throughout the programme as well as documentation of future learning plans and career goals. **Why** Allows you to document your journey through the programme. In job interviews, it can be used to demonstrate a synopsis of your accomplishments and your commitment to personal and professional development. It helps you prepare for the NMC revalidation. **Formative**—submission of certain artefacts or sections of the portfolio at particular points of the course **Summative**—full portfolio expectations

Type of assessment task	Key features and purpose for professional practice
Presentation • **Oral and visual** 	**What** A talk aimed at a peer, professional and/or academic audience about a topic using a set period of time. Often a visual aid is developed and used, e.g., PowerPoint slides, Prezi or poster to support. May be delivered in person, online or by recording. It may be undertaken without a visual prompt, often called a viva voce. **Why** Allows you to demonstrate your knowledge through spoken word and visual materials. You exhibit your communication, time management and, often, your creative and digital literacy skills, too. **Group presentations** also allow you to demonstrate team-working and collaborative skills.
Project 	**What** An extended piece of writing, examining a specific health or nursing phenomenon. It most often addresses an issue identified in placement and proposes areas of research, activities or interventions to develop practice and improve patient outcomes. It's often used as the dissertation. **Why** Allows you to demonstrate your understanding of evidence-based transformational leadership, change and sustainable service improvement.
Reflection 	**What** A piece of writing that uses a reflective model to describe and critically explore a real-life professional, related experience. Typically written in the first person and uses different tenses. May be used for academic and/or practice assessment. **Why** Allows you to demonstrate reflective abilities. Mandated by the NMC (2018e) code, reflection is an essential skill that reviews personal experience and uses critical thinking with the aim of increasing self-awareness and professional knowledge to enhance practice.

Continued

Type of assessment task	Key features and purpose for professional practice
Report	**What** A formal piece of concise writing that documents facts, figures and evidence to explore an issue for a certain audience. It is structured using sections with subheadings and may use bullet points, numbering and figures. Written in the third person and past tense. **Why** Allows you to undertake an in-depth exploration into a health or nursing phenomenon. Enables you to demonstrate investigatory and searching skills and ability to produce findings and recommendations in precise detail. Supports you to exhibit your ability to tailor information to a specific audience. Aside from patient notes, reports are one of the most common types of writing you will undertake as a registered nurse. **Example:** • Exploring a public health issue within a certain population in a particular geographical area for public health commissioners
Research critique	**What** A piece of writing exploring the credibility, robustness and, hence, the effectiveness and usefulness of primary research. Most often written as a structured essay or report or displayed through a poster. **Why** It supports you to demonstrate your research knowledge and its importance for evidence-based practice. Enables you to learn and use critical analysis and evaluative skills.

NMC, Nursing and Midwifery Council; *OSCE,* objective structured clinical examination.

Demonstration of achievement across academic levels

Meeting the learning outcomes or objectives attached to each summative assessment task is mandatory to be successful. Unless the assessment is graded as pass/fail, how well these have been met alongside other measures outlined in the academic and practice assessment criteria will indicate the mark you will be awarded (see 'Assessment criteria' section). As you progress through each part, year and relevant academic level, the expectations of your abilities and, therefore, your achievement, will increase. This will be reflected in the changes in the wording of the learning outcomes or objectives, the amount of independent work you are expected to complete, the length of exams and coursework, as well as the increased complexity of the assessment tasks (Chapter 4).

NMC

THE NMC SAYS

5.6 'Curriculum provides appropriate structure and sequencing that integrates theory and practice at increasing levels of complexity'

The following diagram outlines academic and practice assessment expectations and how they change as students progress through ordinary or honours degrees (Fig. 6.3). Note the common verbs (instruction words) used in learning outcomes or objectives and assessment titles or questions at each level. It is important to know their meaning in order to understand the requirements and be successful.

Assessment organisation

Finally, a useful thing to do to manage assessment expectations is to engage in good organisation (Chapter 2). You will experience multiple assessments, and some exam dates, assignment dates and PAD submission dates may be close together. Ensure you plan ahead for success!

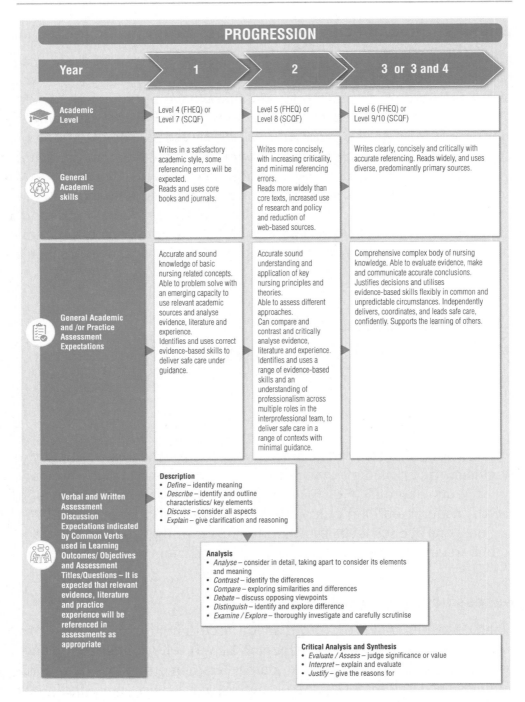

Fig. 6.3   An outline of academic and practice assessment expectations and how they change as students progress through ordinary or honours degrees. *FHEQ*, Frameworks for Higher Education Qualification; *SCQF*, Scottish Credit andQualifications Framework.

- *'Do not leave assessment work to the last minute!*
- *Find your most suitable place to study. Everyone is different, and you may need to test what works for you.*
- *Have a yearly planner on your wall, calendar and/or a diary where you note down all the key assessment dates for your course.*
- *Have a folder and/or notebook (or a notebook with sections) for each module or placement so that you can keep all information and resources for each separately and in one place for easy reference'.*

Beth Dennis and Grace Broughton, second-year child nursing students

ACCESSING SUPPORT AND USING RESOURCES TO PLAN FOR AND COMPLETE ASSESSMENT ACTIVITIES

This section will explore what assessment guidance is available and what resources look like more practically and some key things you can do in preparation and during the completion of each piece of coursework, examination or practice assessment. For detailed information and advice in relation to organisation and planning, see Chapter 2. For key study skills such as reading, note-taking, finding and using literature and referencing, explore Chapter 3, and to understand the skills required for academic writing, review Chapter 4. Here, we will be learning specifically about the importance of assessment briefs, assessment criteria, engaging in formative activities, knowing who can support you and submission processes.

Assessment documents

The assessment brief for an exam or assignment provides an overview of the task at hand, including its nature and objectives, the intended audience and the format or structure of the work. It also outlines the requirements for completion, such as the time limit or word count, referencing style, submission deadlines or exam instructions. By thoroughly understanding the assessment brief, you can ensure you address the task appropriately. Remember, the module or unit learning outcomes are the link between what you learn and how this is assessed in order to evidence your achievement, and there should be some further explanation about these in this document. Take a look at the anatomy of an assessment brief outlined in the following diagram to ensure you understand the importance of each element and what to take note of when preparing and completing your own assessments (Fig. 6.4).

Practice focus. As a nursing student, it is also essential to understand the PAD/ePAD, as it sets out assessment requirements for placement experiences, including professional values, clinical proficiencies (NMC, 2018d) and specific learning outcomes or objectives as agreed with your practice assessor. Like the assessment brief for university-based assessment, ensure that you familiarise yourself with the PAD or ePAD at the start of each placement so you are prepared to demonstrate your ability through various formative and summative assessment tasks and meet the expectations of your practice assessor. The PAD/ePAD is also used to provide feedback on your performance and enables you to reflect on your experiences, facilitating identification of your strengths and weaknesses and planning for ongoing learning and development as you progress throughout the programme.

Assessment criteria

Assessment criteria, sometimes known as grading criteria or marking rubrics, specify the standards and expectations for the quality of work that is being assessed according to the level of study. They provide a clear understanding of the learning outcomes that are being evaluated by the assignment or exam and, therefore, the knowledge, skills and behaviours that are expected to be demonstrated by the student. Consequently, it is the assessment criteria that markers use to pass judgement on a completed assessment and how grades will be allocated, supporting marking to be consistent (see the 'Marking of assessment' section). Most criteria consist of a common framework providing an overall description of different grades and/or an outline of different elements, e.g., knowledge and understanding, organisation of ideas, integrating academic learning and practice, etc., aligned with certain percentages and grade boundaries.

Assessment criteria often vary for each assessment task, so it is vital that you read them at the start of each module or unit of learning. By understanding, studying and writing against the criteria, you will concentrate

Module or unit lead or convener name and contact details

This is the person to contact for general support or information about the assessment

Academic Level

E.g., Level 4

This is the level this assessment is expected to be completed at and will be graded against

Assessment no. and type

E.g., Summative
E.g., CW1: Case Study
EX1: Numeracy
EX2: MCQ anatomy and physiology

This will indicate whether it is a mandatory assessment – summative or optional – formative.

It will also provide an indication of what type of task(s) and what number –e.g. One Coursework element (CW1) OR First Exam (EX1) and Second Exam (EX2) (Multiple choice questions)

Assessment weighting

E.g., CW1 = 100%
EX1 = 25%
EX2 = 75%

If you have more than one assessment per module, this indicates how the marks are allocated. This is important to understand as one assessment may be worth more marks than another and hence demands more time and effort spent on it

Submission or exam time and date

For coursework, this will be the <u>final time</u> you can submit, not the actual time to submit.

If an exam, this is the actual date and time it is undertaken

Target feedback time, date and method

The date to receive your grade and feedback should follow the university academic regulations or indicate if not. It may be oral, written or electronic

Assessment Task

This should include the following information as appropriate:
- Assessment task type e.g., Report, Reflective Essay, Presentation, Unseen time-constrained online exam
- Assignment or Exam title or question
- Word/ time limit of an assignment if written or oral, or length of exam
- A description of the task – this may include topics expected to be included, whether it is an individual or group task
- Structure of the work – this may include word counts/timings for sections and/or expected headings or suggested sections

Learning Outcomes or Objectives

Those that are being assessed should be listed here

Presentation and Referencing Expectations

This should include the following information as appropriate:
- If a submission or cover sheet is required
- Font type and size, line spacing
- Referencing style e.g., Harvard, APA

Fig. 6.4   The anatomy of an assessment brief document.

Continued

Exam Regulations or Submission details

This should include the following information as appropriate:
- Links to university exam regulations and any specific information for your programme or that specific exam
- If an assignment, what format to submit, details of electronic and/or hard (paper) copies, where and how, and who to contact if there are any issues

Help and support

This should highlight what type of support can be accessed, where and who from. This includes any reasonable adjustments.

Any other useful information

This may include information about Academic Integrity/ misconduct and/or maintaining confidentiality. It may also contain instructions of what to do if you have exceptional circumstances which mean you may not be able to sit the exam or submit your work on time.

Assessment Criteria

Some Assessment Briefs may also include the Assessment Criteria (see Assessment Criteria section below). Some universities will provide this on a separate document. For Assessment Criteria using the format outlined below, criterion will be identified which are relevant to the level, assessment and its associated learning outcomes or objectives.

Level 4 Academic level the criteria is written against	0–34% F Fail – not successful	35–39% E Marginal fail	40–49% D or 3rd Satisfactory Pass	50–59% C or 2:2 Good Pass	60–69% B or 2:1 Very Good Pass	70–79% A or 1st Excellent Pass	80–100% A+ or 1st Outstanding Pass
Criterion 1 This should include evidence of:							
Criterion 2 This should include evidence of:							
Etc							

Fig. 6.4, cont'd

your efforts on the most important aspects of the assessment and ensure that you are meeting the required standard to pass. In addition, you can use the criteria to self-evaluate your work before submission, ensuring you've addressed all the required elements. Both the assessment brief and criteria are written by the module or unit lead or convener and checked by another member of staff, often the internal moderator, as well as the external examiner, before you receive them.

Importance of formative activities

As already outlined, formative assessment is optional and aimed at supporting ongoing learning. Formal formative activities, if within theoretical learning, may or may not be graded, but formative activities are predominantly informal and take place regularly in all learning environments. Some you may have come across are:

- Oral presentation of a topic for feedback and feedforward by practice staff
- Creation of assessment plans or concept maps
- Engagement with extracts or whole examples of assessed work in small group activities
- Self-evaluation—e.g., making a draft of your own work before submission, using the assessment criteria that will be used to assess the summative version or engaging in feedback and feedforward from previous summative work to plan actions for improvement (see 'Scrutiny of assessment' section)
- Peer evaluation—e.g., reviewing each other's work

SOCIAL MEDIA
@RakheeLb

'Feedback are invaluable tools and meant to consolidate awareness of strengths and areas to improve, NOT punishing. Shared educational values. Engage positively and support where appropriate'.

You may be tempted to not engage in formative assessment when you review the workload of certain modules or units of learning, but research shows that it is possibly one of the most important activities to support your academic, professional and personal development

(Lewis et al., 2020; Öz and Ordu, 2021; Aase et al., 2022; De Brún et al., 2022). As well as helping summative assessment preparation and subsequent success, benefits for nursing students include:

- Developing topic knowledge and skills as well as critical thinking and problem-solving skills in a safe and supportive environment
- Identifying strengths and weaknesses, which can then be used to guide progress
- Monitoring progress to ensure you are able to meet required standards

NMC

THE NMC SAYS

22.3 'Keep your knowledge and skills up to date, taking part in appropriate and regular learning and professional development activities that aim to maintain and develop your competence and improve your performance'.

Supporting, supervisor and assessor roles

CASE STUDY

Aaliyah, a second-year child nursing student, is struggling to focus on planning her research assignment. She is not enjoying the module and is finding some concepts difficult to grasp. Every time she plans to work on it, she is being easily distracted with other things. She is pretty sure she is the only one finding it difficult and is hesitant to share her feelings.

If you are struggling, it is important to share your concerns to help alleviate feelings of isolation and anxiety and access resources and support services. Sharing experiences and seeking help can also help you develop important communication and problem-solving skills that will be valuable throughout your career. As a nursing student, there are many different roles that can advise and help you with your theoretical and practice assessments. Your university and relevant placement services, as well as specific roles, will be outlined in your programme/course and placement/practice handbooks. There are also mandatory roles set out in the NMC (2018b) standards for supervision and assessment. It is important to understand all the roles available to you and their responsibilities so that you access the correct individual or team and receive support in a timely manner (Fig. 6.5).

Are you confident that you know what you need to do for your current or upcoming theoretical or practice assessments and where, when and how to do it?

If not, make a note of what you need help with and arrange an appointment with the appropriate person or support service.

_____

_____

_____

_____

- *'Start researching and preparing for your assessments as soon as you receive information about them – having time to build on your ideas and gain a proper understanding of the task and the focus is so important*
- *If there is a choice of, or within your, assessment take some time think about your strengths, weaknesses, preferences, and academic or professional skills you may want to enhance further as well as how much time you have to complete each task*
- *Examine your practice assessment document and each assessment brief carefully, make a note/ highlight all the important information*
- *Research topics in depth, gather your literature and evidence-based resources (not through google!), read lots and take notes*
- *Keep track of all the literature and resources that you find – there are some that you will use again and again and this means you can find them more easily*
- *Reach out for support to the appropriate individual or support service if you are finding any aspect of assessment difficult. If you are unsure who that maybe seek guidance from your personal tutor'.*

Beth Dennis and Grace Broughton, second-year child nursing students

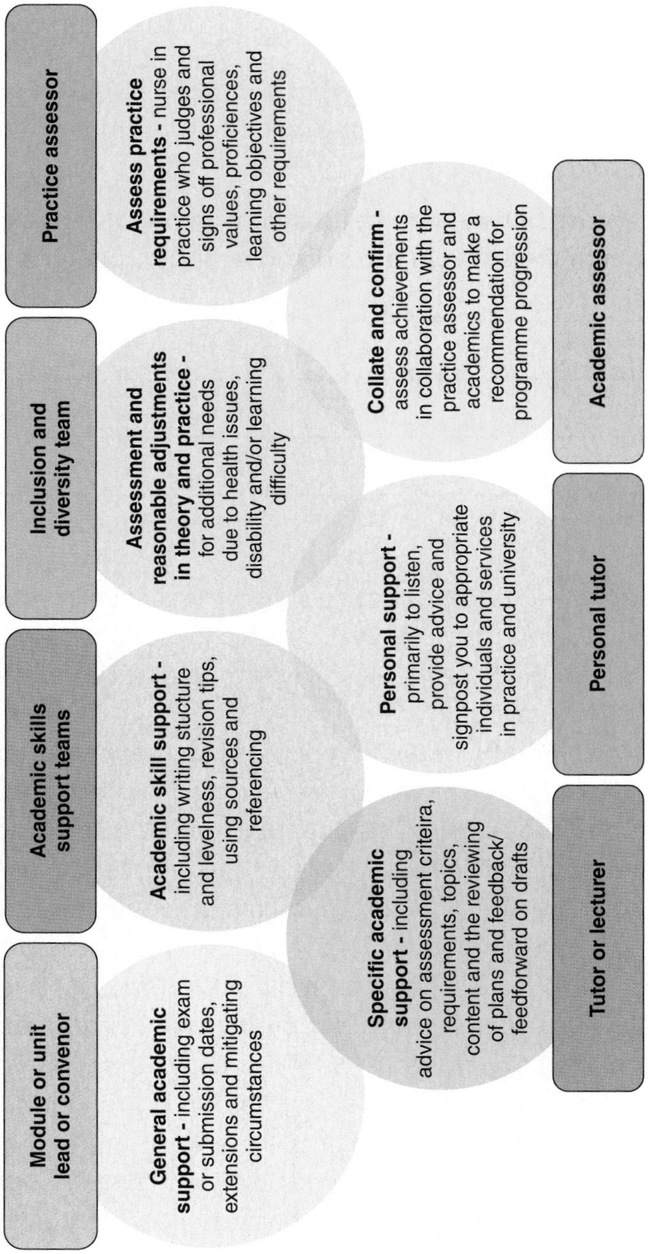

Module or unit lead or convenor

General academic support - including exam or submission dates, extensions and mitigating circumstances

Academic skills support teams

Academic skill support - including writing stucture and levelness, revision tips, using sources and referencing

Inclusion and diversity team

Assessment and reasonable adjustments in theory and practice - for additional needs due to health issues, disability and/or learning difficulty

Practice assessor

Assess practice requirements - nurse in practice who judges and signs off professional values, proficiences, learning objectives and other requirements

Specific academic support - including advice on assessment criteira, requirements, topics, content and the reviewing of plans and feedback/feedforward on drafts

Personal support - primarily to listen, provide advice and signpost you to appropriate individuals and services in practice and university

Collate and confirm - assess achievements in collaboration with the practice assessor and academics to make a recommendation for programme progression

Tutor or lecturer

Personal tutor

Academic assessor

Fig. 6.5   Different roles and services that support you on your assessment journey.

Exceptional circumstances

It is important to be aware of what help you are entitled to when life situations arise that affect your ability to sit an exam, complete an assignment or submit your PAD or ePAD on time or to the best of your ability. Exceptional or extenuating circumstances are those that could not have been prevented or accommodated and can include illness, injury, bereavement, being a victim of a crime, a family crisis or other significant personal issues related to your health, well-being, housing or finances. Seek advice from the identified academic role, and every student union offers independent and impartial advice. The type of support available will vary depending on when the issue occurred and what type of assessment you are completing, so it is important to review your university's guidelines.

Submitting work

For all assessments, whether practice or theoretical, familiarise yourself with the examination rules or submission guidelines as indicated by the assessment brief and programme and placement handbooks. This includes the dates to ensure you attend on the correct day or submit your work on time and in the correct format. When submitting academic assignments, it is essential to understand the importance of originality and academic integrity in your work (Chapter 3). It is likely that your university will use plagiarism detection software such as Turnitin. This tool compares your submission with a vast database of existing work to identify instances of plagiarism. It is possible that a draft Turnitin point or portal will be available to check your work before final submission; if not, Turnitin has a feature called Turnitin Draft Coach (Turnitin, 2023) that supports this as well as other issues that may negatively impact your writing, including structure, grammar, punctuation and spelling. Even if you do not have access to or choose to use these tools, as long as you submit work ahead of the due date, you will still be able to use the resultant similarity report to review your work, identify any issues that may need rectifying and then resubmit. Do this by finding the sections of your work that are highlighted to ensure you have provided a citation, as well as reviewing the list of sources to ensure you have appropriately paraphrased or quoted them in your submission.

Academic assessment

- *'Make a proper plan for each assessment which refers to each learning outcome to ensure you meet these.*
- *As you progress your plan, outline each key point you wish to make, ideas as to how you will do this and add references you will use.*
- *Work on perfecting your referencing.*
- *Always proofread your work by reading aloud and asking someone else to read it for you too'.*

Practice assessment

- *'Attend any additional skills sessions or book out equipment so you can practise observations before you go on placement if your university offers these opportunities.*
- *Have a pocket notebook with key information in such as PEWS/NEWS parameters to keep in your uniform pocket for easy reference.*
- *Take any and all opportunities you can to volunteer in health-care organisations, or spend time with other teams and services while you are on placement'.*

Beth Dennis and Grace Broughton, second-year child nursing students

EVALUATING ACHIEVEMENT AND IMPROVING FOR FUTURE ASSESSMENT

At some point during your nursing studies, it is possible you will receive a grade that you are not happy with, feedback that appears unjust or feedforward you want to understand further. You may feel disappointed, angry or confused, and you may even feel like giving up. These are all reasonable reactions that your university tutors, lecturers, practice supervisors and assessors will understand and want to support you with.

CASE STUDY

'For all my assignments in first year I scraped a pass, and I was so disappointed in myself. It was once I realised that essays don't reflect how I practise that I started to feel more confident. It is important to understand the theory and pass your assignments so you can achieve your degree but don't be hard on yourself if you aren't getting the marks you hoped for. The patients and families won't care if you got 80% or 40% on your essay. They care about how you treat them and how good your nursing skills are'.

Beth Dennis, second-year child nursing student

So, what do you do if you find yourself in this situation? Beth (above) is right to advise not being too hard on yourself. Remind yourself of what you have overcome to get to this point and be proud of what you have achieved so far. A key principle to appreciate is the concept of 'academic judgment' (Higher Education Act, 2004). This means that where academic expert opinion is required and given, such as in the case of assessment, unless there is evidence that procedures have not been followed or a biased decision has been made, this must be respected, and universities' formal complaint or appeals processes cannot interfere with these decisions. More often than not, taking some time to reflect on the information you have received and, if required, having a conversation with the marker, will resolve the issue. Avoid contacting them as soon as you receive your grade, though, to prevent you from communicating in a manner you may regret later—we've all done this when we are upset or angry!

NMC

THE NMC SAYS

8.1 'Respect the skills, expertise and contributions of your colleagues, referring matters to them when appropriate'.

TIP

1. Carefully engage with all the feedback and feedforward you have received. Ask yourself:
   - What is the information telling me?
   - Is the grade really poor? Or is it more that it isn't what I expected or wanted?

2. Refamiliarise yourself with the assessment brief and criteria and reread/listen to the feedback and feedforward. Ask yourself:
   - Have I met the expected requirements for the grade I am expecting?
   - How does my self-assessment compare to the marker's comments?

3. Reflect on what you could have done differently. Ask yourself:
   - Do I understand where I went wrong and how I can improve?

4. If following this, you have any doubts or need clarification about the information you have received, then contact the marker. If it is a small query, this may be resolved easily via email; if not, ask to meet with them to discuss your concerns.

5. If following this, you believe that a mistake has been made and the marker is not in agreement/or is unable to amend
   - If this is before board, your marks are still provisional. Contact the module or unit leader or convener, who may be able to resolve the issue.
   - If this is after board and procedural irregularity has taken place, please refer to the academic appeal process at your university.
   - If you would like guidance or support, contact your student union advice centre.

Practice focus

It is important to note that any concerns regarding assessment in practice must be addressed as soon as possible, rather than waiting until the placement has ended or you have returned to theoretical learning at university. Your placement handbook should provide you with the correct process. These are good tips to follow.

TIP

- Review the assessment process, tasks and criteria as outlined in your PAD to clarify your understanding.
- Raise the concern with your practise assessor to understand what the issue is.
- Escalate the concern if you remain unhappy with the decision made or do not understand the issues by requesting advice from your academic assessor and/or educational lead in the practice area.
- Seek support from your practice supervisor(s), peers and personal tutor as appropriate, as it can be a challenging time.

SOCIAL MEDIA
@NRNpaeds_Ellena

'To be a nurse we have to pass both aspects of the course, placement and theory – therefore correspondence between both areas is crucial... it closes the 'gap' between placement and university'

Nursing students should take ownership of their learning and strive to achieve their best. This includes meeting deadlines, engaging with programme material and formative activities, seeking additional opportunities, accessing support as required as well as engaging with your assessment feedback and feedforward (Burgess and Mellis, 2015; Sadler et al., 2022). In turn, your practice assessors, academic assessors, tutors and lecturers should ensure that you are fairly and reliably assessed. For theoretical assessments, your university will employ various marking, scrutiny and ratification activities to ensure that the grades, feedback and feedforward you receive are true, just and consistent. See the diagram as follows, which outlines the order of these processes (Fig. 6.6).

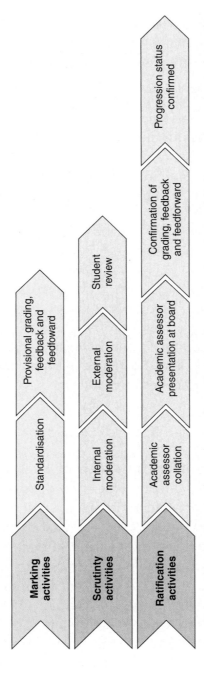

Fig. 6.6 Outline of academic activities that take place once students have completed assessments.

Marking of assessment

For assessments consisting of multiple-choice or short-answer questions, such as written or online quizzes, workbooks or exams, marking is fairly straightforward, as markers will have a clear answer sheet to refer to, or, in some instances, it is completed electronically. For longer-answer exams and other assessment tasks, the work is more nuanced and requires some element of judgement. This is where the assessment criteria come in. Standardisation takes place before academics start marking. The module or unit lead or convener will provide a small sample of submitted exam scripts or assignments to all the markers to assess against the criteria. A meeting is then organised to consider the judgements they have made. This supports all markers in agreeing on the interpretation of the criteria, acceptable standards across grade boundaries and how the feedback and feedforward should be presented.

Scrutiny of assessment

Moderation occurs after the marking has been completed. Internal moderation is undertaken by another nursing academic at the university, who chooses a sample of assessments across all markers and grade boundaries to scrutinise. Primarily, the internal moderator is responsible for ensuring that the markers have applied the marking criteria appropriately and reliably. Any inconsistency or inaccuracy will be raised with the module or unit lead or convener. External moderation is then undertaken by the external examiner, a nursing academic from another university, to ensure that the work is in line with the national norms for the programme of study (Quality Assurance Agency, 2018b).

Feedback and feedforward—and how to use it

Student review is an important part of the scrutiny process. Even if you have no concerns with the grade or feedback/feedforward received, or if it follows formative rather than summative activities, it is always beneficial to proactively engage with it to identify what you did well so as to continue this and what you could improve to ensure ongoing success (Winstone et al., 2017).

SOCIAL MEDIA
@Nix1_87

'As a student, the best feedback I receive is when it involves constructive points, focuses on building/improving practice and allows me key points for reflection to allow me to work through my feelings related to the feedback'

NMC

THE NMC SAYS

9.2 'Gather and reflect on feedback from a variety of sources, using it to improve your practice and performance'.

Creating a mind map of ideas or a checklist of actions or even saving and annotating feedback and feedforward with your reflections and future plans can be useful. Chatting it through with a peer on your course or your personal tutor may be beneficial, too.

Ratification of assessment

For summative assessment, whether theoretical or practice based, results received by students are provisional until they are confirmed by the appropriate board. At most universities, there are two types of boards, which are attended at a minimum by the programme or course lead, module or unit leads or conveners, academic assessors and registry representatives (Quality Assurance Agency, 2018a).

- **Exam or assessment board**, sometimes known as module or programme boards, reviews results and approves marks, determining which students have passed and failed each assessment for the modules or units being presented. These decisions then indicate whether a student can progress or not to the next part of the programme with or without conditions, e.g., retaking assessment(s) and/or placement, completion of deficit placement or theory hours.

Depending on the university's regulations, these recommendations are either submitted to the progression and/or award board for action or are confirmed.

- **Progression and/or award boards** are responsible for verifying a student's eligibility to progress or be awarded. This is determined by whether each student has met expected requirements and confirming their overall grade for that part of study. If at the end of the programme, their award classification is agreed, e.g., 1st, 2:1, 2:2, or 3rd if a bachelor of science or bachelor of science (Hons) degree, or pass, merit or distinction if an integrated masters or postgraduate degree.

Both types of boards also identify any patterns in results that may suggest issues with the module, unit or programme itself. In summary, boards are critical components of assessment processes within your nursing programme, ensuring they are fair and consistent and evaluated using valid and reliable measures. The decision made by these boards determines your progress through and eligibility for your nursing degree.

CONCLUSION

As a nursing student, it is important to understand the principles and practices of assessment in higher education and the nuances within preregistration nursing programmes. As a fundamental aspect, it provides a framework for measuring student knowledge, skill and behaviour and therefore plays a vital role in fitness to practise, fitness for award and, consequently, high-quality patient care. By understanding the different assessment types and tasks, such as theoretical or practice, formative or summative, exam or assignment, students can better prepare to be successful. Furthermore, assessments help identify areas of strength and weakness, enabling students to focus their efforts on areas that require improvement. Hence, it is crucial for nursing students to take assessments seriously and approach them with a positive attitude, using assessment feedback and feedforward as an opportunity for growth and development. Overall, a comprehensive understanding of assessment is crucial for nursing students to achieve academic success and become competent registered nurses.

Now you have finished this chapter. Please make notes on what you have learned.

_____

_____

_____

_____

_____

_____

_____

_____

_____

_____

_____

_____

_____

_____

_____

_____

_____

_____

_____

REFERENCES

Aase, I., Akerjordet, K., Crookes, P., Frøiland, C.T. and Laugaland, K.A. (2022) 'Exploring the formal assessment discussions in clinical nursing education: An observational study', *BMC Nursing*, 21, p. 155. Available at: https://doi.org/10.1186/s12912-022-00934-x.

Biggs, J. (1996) 'Enhancing teaching through constructive alignment', *Higher Education*, 32(3), pp. 347–364. Available at: https://doi.org/10.1007/BF00138871.

Burgess, A. and Mellis, C. (2015) 'Feedback and assessment for clinical placements: Achieving the right balance', *Advances in Medical Education and Practice*, 6, pp. 373–381. Available at: https://doi.org/10.2147/AMEP.S77890.

Culha, I. (2019) 'Active learning methods used in nursing education', *Journal of Pedagogical Research*, 3(2), pp. 74–86.

De Brún, A., Rogers, L., Drury, A. and Gilmore, B. (2022) 'Evaluation of a formative peer assessment in research methods teaching using an online platform: a mixed methods pre-post study', *Nurse Education Today*, 108, p. 105166. Available at: https://doi.org/10.1016/j.nedt.2021.105166.

Department of Health and Social Care (2016) *Nursing degree apprenticeship: factsheet*, *GOV.UK*. Available at: https://www.gov.uk/government/publications/nursing-degree-apprenticeships-factsheet/nursing-degree-apprenticeship-factsheet (Accessed: 14 March 2023).

Duers, L.E. and Brown, N. (2009) 'An exploration of student nurses' experiences of formative assessment', *Nurse Education Today*, 29(6), pp. 654–659. Available at: https://doi.org/10.1016/j.nedt.2009.02.007.

Equality Act 2010 c.15. Available at: http://www.legislation.gov.uk/ukpga/2010/15/contents (Accessed: 9 October 2022).

Higher Education Act 2004, c. 8. Statute Law Database. Available at: https://www.legislation.gov.uk/ukpga/2004/8/part/2/2004-12-01 (Accessed: 20 January 2023).

Hunt, L.A., McGee, P., Gutteridge, R. and Hughes, M. (2012) 'Assessment of student nurses in practice: a comparison of theoretical and practical assessment results in England', *Nurse Education Today*, 32(4), pp. 351–355. Available at: https://doi.org/10.1016/j.nedt.2011.05.010.

Institute for Apprenticeships and Technical Education (2022) *Registered nurse degree (NMC 2018)*, Institute for Apprenticeships and Technical Education. Available at: https://www.instituteforapprenticeships.org/apprenticeship-standards/registered-nurse-degree-nmc-2018-v1-1 (Accessed: 11 December 2022).

Ipsos (2022) *Ipsos Veracity Index 2022*, Ipsos. Available at: https://www.ipsos.com/en-ie/ipsos-veracity-index-2022 (Accessed: 23 November 2022).

Kivunja, C. (2015) 'Why students don't like assessment and how to change their perceptions in 21st century pedagogies', *Creative Education*, 06(20), p. 2117. Available at: https://doi.org/10.4236/ce.2015.620215.

Koh, L.C. (2010) 'Academic staff perspectives of formative assessment in nurse education', *Nurse Education in Practice*, 10(4), pp. 205–209. Available at: https://doi.org/10.1016/j.nepr.2009.08.007.

Lewis, P., Hunt, L., Ramjan, L.M., Daly, M., O'Reilly, R. and Salamonson, Y. (2020) 'Factors contributing to undergraduate nursing students' satisfaction with a video assessment of clinical skills', *Nurse Education Today*, 84, p. 104244. Available at: https://doi.org/10.1016/j.nedt.2019.104244.

Mills, A., Ryden, J. and Knight, A. (2020) 'Juggling to find balance: hearing the voices of undergraduate student nurses', *British Journal of Nursing*, 29(15), pp. 897–903. Available at: https://doi.org/10.12968/bjon.2020.29.15.897.

Nieminen, J.H. (2022) 'Assessment for Inclusion: rethinking inclusive assessment in higher education', *Teaching in Higher Education*, 27(1), pp. 1–19. Available at: https://doi.org/10.1080/13562517.2021.2021395.

Nursing and Midwifery Council (2018a) *Standards for pre-registration nursing programmes*. Available at: https://www.nmc.org.uk/standards/standards-for-nurses/standards-for-pre-registration-nursing-programmes/ (Accessed: 6 November 2022).

Nursing and Midwifery Council (2018b) *Standards for student supervision and assessment*. Available at: https://www.nmc.org.uk/standards-for-education-and-training/standards-for-student-supervision-and-assessment/ (Accessed: 13 November 2022).

Nursing and Midwifery Council (2018c) *Standards framework for nursing and midwifery education*. Available at: https://www.nmc.org.uk/standards-for-education-and-training/standards-framework-for-nursing-and-midwifery-education/ (Accessed: 13 November 2022).

Nursing and Midwifery Council (2018d) *Standards of proficiency for registered nurses*. Available at: https://www.nmc.org.uk/standards/standards-for-nurses/standards-of-proficiency-for-registered-nurses/ (Accessed: 3 January 2023).

Nursing and Midwifery Council (2018e) *The code. Professional standards of practice and behaviour for nurses, midwives and nursing associates*. London: Nursing and Midwifery Council. Available at: https://www.nmc.org.uk/globalassets/sitedocuments/nmc-publications/nmc-code.pdf (Accessed: 13 November 2022).

Öz, G.Ö. and Ordu, Y. (2021) 'The effects of web based education and Kahoot usage in evaluation of the knowledge and skills regarding intramuscular injection among nursing students', *Nurse Education Today*, 103, p. 104910. Available at: https://doi.org/10.1016/j.nedt.2021.104910.

Poindexter, K., Hagler, D. and Lindell, D. (2015) 'Designing authentic assessment: Strategies for nurse educators', *Nurse Educator*, 40(1), pp. 36–40. Available at: https://doi.org/10.1097/NNE.0000000000000091.

Quality Assurance Agency (2014) *Qualifications frameworks*. Available at: https://www.qaa.ac.uk/quality-code/qualifications-frameworks (Accessed: 6 November 2022).

Quality Assurance Agency (2018a) *Assessment*. Available at: https://www.qaa.ac.uk/quality-code/advice-and-guidance/assessment (Accessed: 6 November 2022).

Quality Assurance Agency (2018b) *External expertise*. Available at: https://www.qaa.ac.uk/the-quality-code/advice-and-guidance/external-expertise. (Accessed: 6 November 2022).

Sadler, I., Reimann, N. and Sambell, K. (2022) 'Feedforward practices: a systematic review of the literature', *Assessment & Evaluation in Higher Education*, 48(3), pp. 305-20. Available at: https://doi.org/10.1080/02602938.2022.2073434.

Scott, I.M. (2020) 'Beyond "driving": The relationship between assessment, performance and learning', *Medical Education*, 54(1), pp. 54–59. Available at: https://doi.org/10.1111/medu.13935.

Scottish Credit and Qualifications Framework (2022) *Scottish Credit and Qualifications Framework, Scottish Credit and Qualifications Framework.* Available at: https://scqf.org.uk/about-the-framework/interactive-framework/ (Accessed: 11 December 2022).

Turnitin (2023) *How to use Draft Coach.* Available at: https://help.turnitin.com/integrity/student/draft-coach/using-draft-coach.htm (Accessed: 18 March 2023).

Winstone, N.E., Nash, R.A., Parker, M. and Rowntree, J. (2017) 'Supporting learners' agentic engagement with feedback: A systematic review and a taxonomy of recipience processes', *Educational Psychologist*, 52(1), pp. 17–37. Available at: https://doi.org/10.1080/00461520.2016.1207538.

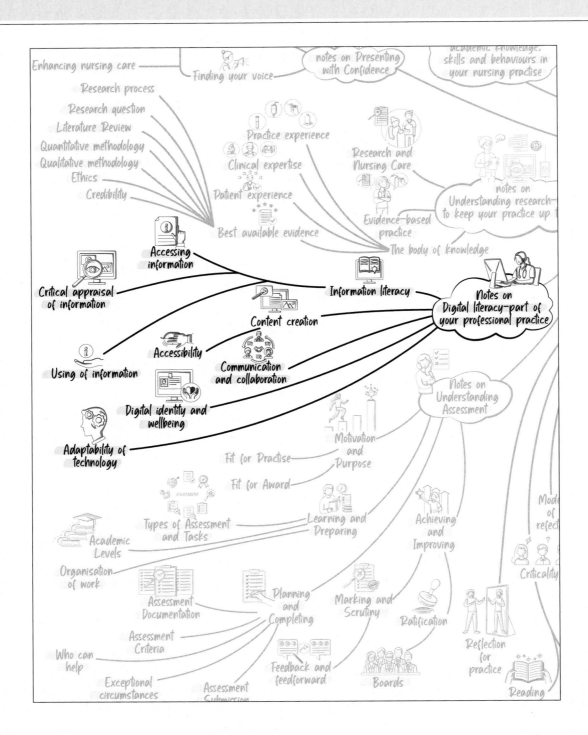

NOTES ON DIGITAL LITERACY— PART OF YOUR PROFESSIONAL PRACTICE

Cathryn Peppard (she/her)

INTRODUCTION

This chapter will explore the fundamental aspects of digital literacy and its implications for your role as a future nurse. There are several definitions of digital literacy (Health Education England, no date; Jisc, 2014), but all of them centre on the same principle: that being digitally literate is having the skills to learn, live and work in the digital environment. There are a lot of different skills and technologies that make up the digital environment, but you aren't expected to know all of them. Instead, you should think about being digitally literate as having an individual or personal benchmark for success, ensuring you have the skills you need to get the most out of your day-to-day life, studies and career.

One example of a day-to-day digital skill would be digital photography. These days, most of us have a smartphone, which we use to take pictures of family and friends, stunning sunsets or something that catches our eye when out and about. Using a smartphone to take photos is a form of digital literacy, as we are using digital technology to carry out this day-to-day task.

Our ability with specific digital skills will vary, and we don't need to be an expert in every area. For some people, taking a digital photo might be their limit and enough for their everyday lives. Other people might want to share their photos more widely, so they will need to use other digital skills to achieve this, such as uploading the photo to social media, applying a filter and including some tags.

Digital literacy is progressive: we gain skills over time, and they will evolve as technology does. Rather than viewing being digitally literate as a set of specific tasks or technologies we want to use, it's helpful to think of it as having the confidence to tackle the unexpected and to adapt to change as it happens. By delving into the realm of digital literacy, you will gain an understanding of its direct relevance to your profession and how it can enhance your capabilities in providing healthcare. We will also uncover the benefits that digital literacy brings and the opportunities to harness its potential. Moreover, this chapter will guide you on effectively utilising technology in alignment with your responsibilities as a nursing professional, ensuring that you can navigate the digital landscape with confidence and skill.

EMBRACING DIGITAL LITERACY: A VITAL SKILLSET FOR FUTURE NURSES

In this section, we will explore the significance of improving your digital literacy skills for your nursing degree and future career.

> **What digital literacies or skills do you require in your day-to-day life? What skills do you think you might need in your nursing career?**
>
> _____
>
> _____
>
> _____
>
> _____
>
> _____

There are two ways that improving your digital literacy skills will be important to your nursing degree and career in the next few years. Firstly, they can help you to study more effectively, saving you time and effort when it comes to completing assignments. Secondly, being digitally literate will help you maximise the benefits of technology for you and your patients and improve healthcare outcomes.

The Nursing and Midwifery Council (NMC) (2018) code doesn't have an explicit section about digital technology, but the principles of the code can only be upheld if they are applied to all parts of your life, including the digital.

NMC

THE NMC SAYS

6.1 'Make sure that any information or advice given is evidence-based including information relating to using any health and care products or services'.

7.3 'Use a range of verbal and non-verbal communication methods, and consider cultural sensitivities, to better understand and respond to people's personal and health needs'.

For example, to fulfil elements of the NMC (2018) code listed above, you may need to use online journals and digital databases to access the best available evidence. Additionally, you may need to use email, social media or design patient information using digital tools to be able to communicate clearly. These are all digital activities that will enable you to follow the NMC (2018) code and deliver excellent nursing care.

Many employers and your professional body, the Royal College of Nursing (RCN), also have expectations around digital skills being part of a nurse's skill set. The RCN's (2018) 'Every nurse an e-nurse' report sets out a vision for the future of nursing, where every nurse has the skills required to practise effectively using digital tools. The RCN cited 'better outcomes for patients... better experiences for staff... [and] more efficient ways of working' (2018, p 5) as the benefits of ensuring the future workforce is digitally literate. Health Education England (2018), which is now part of NHS England, set out their own ambitions for nursing and digital, which envision a digitally connected and efficient profession.

Digital literacy is rapidly becoming a core skill, alongside any other part of nursing practice.

Perhaps at this point, you feel convinced, or maybe you didn't need convincing to begin with. You are ready for the next steps and to start building your digital skills. Hopefully, you have already taken the time described to reflect and identify some core areas you want to work at. Those reflections are useful to look back on and to help you see how this might change over time, as well as to enable you to put a learning plan in place to improve these skills. The rest of the chapter will break down specific elements of digital literacy and suggest things you can do to build your skills and confidence.

There are multiple different digital literacy frameworks that exist (Health Education England, 2018; Jisc, 2014). Each framework has its own perspective, but the essential components tend to be the same across them all. The key areas of focus tend to be information literacy (a topic in its own right, but a key component of digital literacy), communication and collaboration, content creation, digital identity and well-being and adaptability (see Fig. 7.1). We're going to look briefly at each of these and see how they apply to our practice and studies.

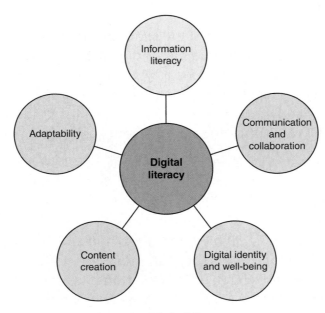

Fig. 7.1   Digital literacy.

INFORMATION LITERACY

Information literacy deals with how we find, access, critically appraise and use information (Chartered Institute of Library and Information Professionals, 2018; UNESCO, 2023). It has become a central part of digital literacy, as many of us now use the internet to find and access information. In addition, the internet has altered how we publish information with anyone able to write a blog post, contribute to Wikipedia or make a webpage. This has been both an equaliser for information, allowing more people with expert knowledge or lived experience to share their learning, but at the same time, it means that it is very easy to promote false or inaccurate information. Critical awareness and good information literacy can help us navigate information in the digital space.

Finding and accessing information

When looking for information, it's important to consider what it is you are looking for. Are you looking for a healthcare report or, perhaps, statistics on how common type 2 diabetes is in the general population? Maybe you need an introduction to wound care and best practice guidance on how to treat pressure sores. There are a variety of online search engines or databases that can be helpful, but they have their strengths and weaknesses, depending on what you are looking for.

To begin with, popular search engines like Google are great tools for quickly finding a wide range of information, especially grey literature. As outlined in Chapter 3, grey literature includes information, reports or statistics published by government bodies, charitable organisations or international entities like the World Health Organization. This type of information is often available online, and search engines excel at locating it. On the other hand, when searching for academic articles and research papers typically found in journals, specialised databases prove to be invaluable. These focus on specific disciplines such as nursing or healthcare, and gather high-quality journals related to those subjects. By using databases, you can efficiently search across numerous credible sources and access evidence-based information for patient care. Access to these databases typically requires a login, which can often be obtained through your university library, placement, workplace library or a specialist library like at the

RCN if you are a member. In addition, training on how to use the databases is often available through the library. There is a growing trend to publish articles and information as 'open access', which means that you do not need a library login to be able to download for free. Google Scholar, the academic version of Google, is usually very good at locating open-access versions of articles when they are available, and it can also be worth searching Google Scholar if your library does not have access to a specific article you may have found during a search. Please review Chapter 3, which discusses databases and literature searching in detail.

TIP

Many online eBook platforms, databases or eJournals will have accessibility functions like speech to text or the ability for you to change the font or background. Explore the help or accessibility pages to find out the specifics for the resource you are using.

Critical appraisal

Whether you have found the information through Google, a database or by recommendation, you need to critically appraise the information to check that it is reliable and well evidenced. This can be especially important with online information, as it is incredibly easy for people to publish information that looks credible, even if it's not. We've seen this during the COVID-19 pandemic where inaccurate information was shared about the virus, how it was spread and the vaccination. Being able to think critically about information helps us assess its reliability and ensures that we are using the best available evidence (see Chapter 5 for further information about critical thinking reading). Remember, the NMC code (2018) requires you to practise with the best available evidence, so it is crucial you seek out high-quality evidence and critically appraise it yourself.

NMC

THE NMC SAYS

6.2 'Maintain the knowledge and skills you need for safe and effective practice'.

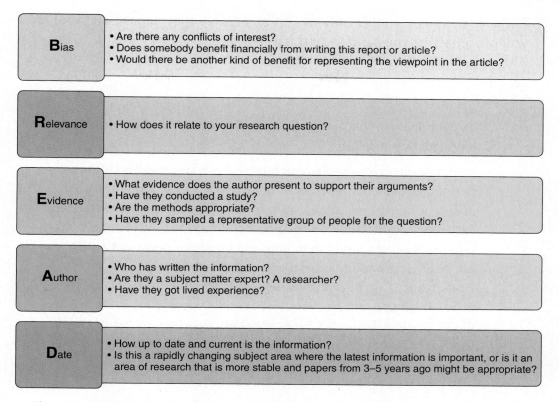

Bias
- Are there any conflicts of interest?
- Does somebody benefit financially from writing this report or article?
- Would there be another kind of benefit for representing the viewpoint in the article?

Relevance
- How does it relate to your research question?

Evidence
- What evidence does the author present to support their arguments?
- Have they conducted a study?
- Are the methods appropriate?
- Have they sampled a representative group of people for the question?

Author
- Who has written the information?
- Are they a subject matter expert? A researcher?
- Have they got lived experience?

Date
- How up to date and current is the information?
- Is this a rapidly changing subject area where the latest information is important, or is it an area of research that is more stable and papers from 3–5 years ago might be appropriate?

Fig. 7.2 BREAD—a simple acronym for five things to think about when selecting information.

There are resources that help you with critical appraisal. An easy-to-remember checklist that's useful for quick, initial assessments is the acronym BREAD (Bedford, 2018); see Fig. 7.2:

SOCIAL MEDIA

@KaaraCalma

'Critical appraisal of evidence is an important transferable skill that #Nurses need. This is not only for when we use evidence to inform practice, but also when educating patients on how to seek & use reliable information amidst a plethora of misleading resources'.

There are more complex critical appraisal tools that might be useful as you progress in your studies and career.

 TIP

You might find the following resources helpful when getting started with critical appraisal:

- Understanding Health Research provides a step-by-step introduction to appraising a research article in a bit more depth, but still aimed at beginners: https://www.understandinghealthresearch.org/
- Dr Greenhalgh's book on reading academic papers is widely cited and used across multiple health and medical courses; it covers every aspect of understanding and assessing papers:
  Greenhalgh, T. (2019) *How To Read a Paper: The Basics of Evidence-Based Medicine and Healthcare*. 6th edn. Oxford: John Wiley & Sons.
- CASP (Critical Appraisal Skills Program) provides in-depth checklists for different kinds of evidence papers: https://casp-uk.net/casp-tools-checklists/
  https://www.understandinghealthresearch.org/

Using information

Once we have found the evidence we need, we need to be able to apply it to either practical use or for our assignments. When we use research and evidence in our writing, we need to ensure we acknowledge our sources correctly. This demonstrates that we have read widely on our subject and have considered the findings of previous research or thinking, and it adds authority to our arguments. I won't cover referencing in detail here—please see Chapter 3 for this—but in a chapter about digital literacy, it would be remiss not to mention some of the digital tools that can help.

Referencing is something that can cause stress and anxiety amongst even seasoned writers. A reference manager allows you to collect, organise and then cite your reading as you go along. There are several types of reference managers that are available, varying from paid for to free. Some are entirely web or cloud based, so you use them through your internet browser, whereas others are software you download. Your university may have a subscription to one of the paid-for reference managers—examples include EndNote and RefWorks—so it is worth asking. If you don't have access to one of the paid-for reference managers, then Zotero offers an entirely free desktop option. However, if you need something simple that you can access anywhere, ZoteroBib (2022) has everything you need. ZoteroBib is perfect for creating reference lists and in-text citations, and you don't need to download anything, meaning you can access it on any computer or even your smartphone.

CONTENT CREATION

These days, content tends to be created digitally. When writing essays or reports, you are likely to be using Word or Pages (Apple's equivalent) rather than writing them by hand. This content is known as 'born digital', as it started its existence through a digital format. Being able to create and edit content digitally is a crucial skill for any student, and hopefully, it should be able to make things easier at the same time.

It helps to think of content creation as anything original you produce. This could be patient notes, an essay, an email or a tweet; these are all examples of creating digital content. Familiarising yourself with some basic programs like the Microsoft Office suite, or the Google equivalent, is a good idea, as Word, Excel and PowerPoint are used everywhere. They will build your confidence with branching out to other tools or software, and there are plenty of how-to help videos online to get you started. Many, if not all, universities offer a free download of Microsoft Office tools or provide access to their online versions through an Office 365 account. Your university librarian or student centre will be able to help direct you to where you can access these tools.

When communicating digitally, you have the option to think differently about how you present ideas. Depending on your assignment guidelines, you may be able to create an online poster or interactive presentation rather than a standard PowerPoint (see Chapter 6).

Canva (2023) lets you create infographics or visual-based content for presentations or social media. Mentimeter (2023) allows you to create interactive slides where you can invite audience participation, or you could try something like Kahoot! (2023) to run a quiz for your classmates. Depending on what you want to do, there will probably be a tool that can help. Reaching out on Twitter and asking other nursing students will bring back lots of suggestions, or searching for 'free presentation tools' will provide options, too.

Creating content is about more than just designing or producing the content; you also need to plan and manage your time as you do it. Mind-mapping tools can be great when planning an essay or project. Miro (2023) and Canva (2023) are two examples that let you create free mind maps, and Miro offers options for you to share your mind map collaboratively (see Chapter 11 for other examples). Sometimes it can be hard to concentrate or focus to meet deadlines, and there are some great digital options to help with that, too. The Pomodoro technique (outlined in Chapter 2) can help you focus, and there are countless timers online designed around it, but my favourite is Pomofocus (2023). If you need something a little more creative, or to help you ignore your phone, then an app like Forest (2023) might work. It grows a tree whilst you work, but if you leave before the timer is up, the tree will die, so you are encouraged to keep focused. See Fig. 7.3 for a round up of tools outlined here.

Documents and spreadsheets	Presentations	Mind mapping	Staying focused
• Microsoft Office - Has tools for creating documents (Word), spreadsheets (Excel) and presentations (PowerPoints). Can be shared. • Google - a free set of tools that let you create documents (Docs), spreadsheets (Sheets) and presentations (Slides). These are easily shareable.	• PowerPoint - A Microsoft Office tool commonly used to create presentations. • Slides - a Google tool used to create presentations, similar to PowerPoint. • Canva (2023) - helps create infographics or visual content. • Mentimeter (2023) - interactive slides. • Kahoot (2023) - creates quizzes for presentations.	• Miro (2023) - collaborative mind maps. • Canva (2023) - mind maps you can download to share.	• Pomofocus (2023) - a timer to help you with the Pomodoro technique. • Forest (2023) - an app for your phone that encourages you to focus for a set amount of time.

Fig. 7.3   A round-up of tools.

Accessibility when creating content

Technology's strength lies in its ability to create a more accessible environment for everyone. However, this relies on those who use technology to participate in making it accessible. When we create digital content, we should think about using the features of whatever technology we're using to maximise accessibility. For example, when inserting images in documents or posting them online, there is usually the option to add alt text that enables people with screen readers to understand what the image depicts. Likewise, if you are adding links to your text, then think about what will be read out to someone using a screen reader. You should avoid pasting the whole link or putting text like 'click here', which doesn't indicate to someone using a screen reader where the link will take them.

The fonts and colours we use can equally be important to ensure something is easily read by someone with colour blindness or with a specific learning difficulty like dyslexia. Generally, a sans serif font such as Arial or Calibri is best, as they do not have unnecessary flicks and design features that make it difficult to read. You could even use a font like Dyslexie, which has been specifically designed for readers with dyslexia to avoid the switching and swapping of letters that some people with dyslexia experience. Colours are important, as for some individuals certain colours can cause visual distortion, or, in the case of someone who experiences colour blindness, they may not be able to read it at all. Avoiding red on green or green on red helps with the most common colour blindness. Using a buff yellow background can help some readers with a learning difficulty, as black text on white can be dazzling and difficult to read (see Chapter 11).

Accessibility matters, as making changes to be more accessible is a way that you can treat other people with respect. Using these features will benefit colleagues or patients when sharing information. The NMC code (2018) also states that nurses should ensure that people are treated with dignity and have their communication needs met. By ensuring your digital communication methods are accessible, you are preemptively meeting a communication need and upholding their dignity by ensuring they do not need to ask for basic requirements to be met.

NMC

THE NMC SAYS

1.1 'Treat people with kindness, respect and compassion'.

1.3 'Avoid making assumptions and recognise diversity and individual choice'.

1.5 'Respect and uphold people's human rights' and 'take reasonable steps to meet people's language and communication needs, providing, wherever possible, assistance to those who need help to communicate their own or other people's needs'.

We've discussed access ability a few times in this chapter. What are some of the ways you can ensure your digital content is accessible? Are there accessibility features you will explore for your own benefit?

_____

_____

_____

_____

_____

COMMUNICATION AND COLLABORATION

Digital technology has opened new ways for us to connect with friends, family and colleagues. Whilst it has the obvious benefits of faster communication through emails, messenger services like WhatsApp or Telegram, and online meetings, it has also created opportunities for us to collaborate and work together simultaneously. Like much of technology, it's not about using all of it or using everything in the same way. Thinking about your message, who needs to see it and how best to communicate it will help you pick the right tool for the job. Many people find that they receive too many emails, so you might want to consider using email for when you have a formal message to communicate to multiple people, whereas a Teams message or WhatsApp group might be better for smaller groups with a more informal purpose.

Social media comes up regularly throughout this chapter because it has opened so many doors as a digital tool, and communication is one of its biggest benefits. Social media has been used successfully by multiple healthcare professionals and services to communicate with patients, the public and with their peers. This was seen strongly during the COVID-19 pandemic, where many healthcare professionals took to platforms like Twitter, Instagram, TikTok and YouTube to communicate critical information about the COVID-19 vaccines. Using interactive platforms allowed the public to ask questions or raise concerns about the vaccine with a healthcare professional and have some of their concerns alleviated. It was also used to communicate essential public health messages such as how the virus was transmitted and steps the public could take to prevent catching COVID-19.

As well as using social media to reach out to the public and patients, many nurses use platforms like Twitter as part of their continuing professional development (CPD). There are active nursing communities throughout Twitter that offer support to fellow nurses and run regular 'tweetchats' on different aspects of nursing. The most well-known and active UK nursing community on Twitter is @WeNurses, which has multiple other accounts that cover a variety of nursing specialties, including @WeStudentNurse. The WeNurses accounts also have hashtags you can follow or search for to see messages surrounding a specific topic like #WeStNs for nursing students. Getting involved in a tweetchat can count to your revalidation CPD hours once you are qualified.

It is important to remember that privacy and patient confidentiality still need to be respected online. If you are going to use social media or forums for reflection or to share your experiences, be careful with anonymising any information. Avoid using specific details that might make a patient identifiable, perhaps concentrate more on what you learnt and how you were impacted by the experience. The NMC (2019) has guidance that outlines in detail how the NMC code applies to social media, and it is worth familiarising yourself with it if you are a social media user.

NMC

THE NMC SAYS

5.1 'Respect a person's right to privacy in all aspects of their care'.

5.2 'Make sure that people are informed about how and why information is used and shared by those who will be providing care'.

In the last few years, online meeting software like Teams, Zoom and WebEx has become widespread, as the pandemic changed how many of us communicated. Telehealth, where nurses, doctors or other health-care practitioners meet with patients over the phone or via video conferencing systems took off with 36% of general practice appointments being via phone or video in October 2020 compared to 15% in February 2020 (Quality Watch, 2020). Education moved almost entirely online during the pandemic, and whilst face-to-face teaching has resumed across all sectors, the impact of millions of people needing to use video conferencing and other technology will remain. You may even be taking some of your lectures or modules online using tools such as Blackboard Collaborate. Getting familiar with the fundamentals of any video conferencing system will be useful, as you learn the basic features and etiquette around online meetings, especially as many of these will be transferable across systems.

Working online has lots of benefits as a student, particularly when carrying out group work. Being able to meet up online can save lots of time when your group may be out on placements or travelling from different locations. There are lots of apps and websites you can use to work collaboratively on projects. Tools like Google Docs and Google Slides allow you to share the same project and work on it simultaneously. Microsoft Office has similar functions with its OneDrive and its app versions of software like Word and PowerPoint. There are other collaborative tools that might be useful when working on projects. Padlet (no date) works as a digital corkboard where you can put 'sticky notes' to share ideas and make plans. Trello (2023) allows you to create project boards with to-do lists and actions, ideal for knowing who is working on what or even managing your own time. Most meeting software lets you share screens so you can discuss ideas and see what someone else is doing or start a whiteboard that you can all contribute to.

DIGITAL IDENTITY AND WELL—BEING

As a nursing student, you represent the profession in your online interactions as well as your day-to-day interactions. Whilst you might use social media in a personal capacity, you still have a responsibility to uphold the NMC code (2018), and any breaches of the code online are as serious as if they happened in real life. With this in mind, it is important to consider your digital identity and how to look after yourself online.

Digital identity

The internet is difficult to avoid using altogether, as we are often required to use it to fill out forms, register for services or carry out a task for our jobs. You may not participate in online forums or social media, but every interaction you have online is still forming part of your digital identity. The data we submit to websites, such as our names, date of birth, where we live and photos, all build up a picture of who we are online. It is important that we protect this information and consider how we present ourselves digitally, as this can often be linked back to who we are in our day-to-day lives.

As the internet often becomes a necessary tool for us to participate fully in society, it is useful to think about how and why you want to use the internet, as this can determine how you want to present yourself online. It can also indicate the best ways for you to engage online and narrow down the right platforms for you to interact digitally.

How do you currently use the internet? Think about the types of websites or apps you use on a daily basis. Why are you on those platforms?

_____

_____

_____

_____

_____

By participating in life digitally, we need to consider our personas online and how we want to present ourselves. This includes when we want to use a website or app personally or professionally, as that will impact the kind of information we choose to share. Many of us try to present an idealised version of ourselves and generally promote the positive aspects of our lives. There is nothing wrong with presenting a positive version of yourself, but it helps to try and be as authentic to yourself as possible, especially as there will be people who know both versions of you, and you want people to recognise who you are in each of them.

Whether you choose to use a certain website personally or professionally, you should assume that the widest possible audience will see your profile and what you post. It may seem obvious to state, but you shouldn't post anything online that you wouldn't say or share with somebody in real life. There have been many incidents of people posting 'jokes' or sharing pictures of a night out or controversial viewpoints which have been seen by work colleagues or professional peers and led to them losing their jobs. Whether it happens online or in person, you are still accountable to the NMC (2018) code and should act accordingly.

SOCIAL MEDIA
@PUNC21_jordan

'Digital professionalism should always be in the back of your mind. Professionalism in the public eye does not stop when you clock out of work and has to be maintained as you are a role model for the community. #PUNC21 #NRS410 @WeNurses @WeStudentNurse #DAY3 #WeStNs #NMCCouncil'

Online privacy is an issue that affects everyone. Almost all social media platforms have privacy settings that allow you to limit who sees your posts or can access your profile. They all work to varying degrees, with some sites allowing you to set 'circles' or groups of people who can access specific posts, pictures or content based on how you mark the content when you post it. This can be a way to balance your professional and personal identities online, allowing a limited group of friends access to more personal content. You may also want to vary this platform by platform. For example, Twitter is a popular platform for nurses to engage with each other professionally, so you may want to post more professional content on Twitter and save personal content and photos for Instagram, where interactions tend to be shorter and less conversational.

Well-being

Whilst there are lots of benefits with digital technology, it is important to set boundaries and make sure to protect your well-being. Setting a boundary could be as simple as only checking your email account at set times of the day or limiting the amount of time you spend on social media platforms. Turning notifications off on the app versions of your online accounts can be a great way to set a boundary, as you are not interrupted throughout the day with notifications designed to get you to log back in. It means that you are using technology on your terms and when you want to engage with it.

In the last few years, there has been a rise in cyberbullying and countless stories about how social media can affect our mental health. If you do experience negative behaviour or notice that certain tags or content is disturbing you, then many websites have the option for you to block certain keywords or hashtags. If it is a specific account or person, you should be able to block that account to stop seeing messages from it and block that account from contacting you. If blocking feels too extreme, then many online platforms allow you to mute certain users. This means you can choose to access their content, and they can still view yours, but their posts won't appear in your feed, and you can take a break from that user.

Importantly, if you feel that another user on any kind of digital platform has moved into harassment or bullying, you should document the content with screenshots to avoid them being deleted later, and raise these concerns immediately. You can do this through the online platform itself, but if you feel that the abuse is coming from someone you know professionally, whether a patient, colleague or another student, then speak to your placement or university. In certain cases, it may be necessary to report the behaviour to the police, particularly if you experience an interaction that feels threatening.

CASE STUDY

Leonie was a children and young people's (CYP) nursing student during the pandemic. Due to the lockdowns in the United Kingdom and the government advice for people to stay at home, many nursing students had their education radically change overnight with lectures and learning moving online. This had some positive impacts for Leonie, such as being able to access webinars and conferences without needing to travel, but it had drawbacks too, such as having access to large amounts of learning opportunities which could be overwhelming at times.

Recognising the opportunities digital technology offered for learning and professional development, Leonie became involved with a national online peer support group on Twitter called the Children and Young People's Student Nurse Network (@CYPStNN). The network is staffed by nursing students who volunteer to tweet about their recent learning by sharing information such as interesting articles, YouTube videos, personal reflections or national guidelines. They also have regular tweetchats, which encourage discussion and learning. This had multiple benefits; firstly, it helped Leonie with revision by teaching her knowledge to an audience, which cemented the learning. Secondly, it benefited other CYP nursing students by sharing information and resources which provided learning opportunities. Lastly, it helped Leonie think about how to curate her professional identity on Twitter, such as ensuring that her tweets were evidence based and accurate.

Leonie's experiences with Twitter continued during her time volunteering with the COVID-19 vaccination effort. Many healthcare professionals were using the hashtag #GetVaccinatedNow to

CASE STUDY—cont'd

encourage the public to take up the COVID-19 vaccine. Leonie tweeted out her reasons for getting vaccinated and encouraged others to do the same. Later that day, she came back to dozens of replies from people, some of which were angry and nasty in tone. Leonie was able to recognise that, as a nursing student, it was important to remain professional and tweet in accordance with the NMC code whilst, at the same time, recognising the need to protect her own well-being. Following advice from her workplace, Leonie did not engage with these commenters and turned the comments off for that tweet, which stopped further replies. A university lecturer who saw the comments on Twitter also reached out to offer advice and support.

Reflecting on the incident, Leonie felt that the hashtag came across as a demand statement and that could provoke strong opinions in people. If she were to tweet something similar in the future, she would use a more encouraging hashtag to foster constructive discussion. As Leonie was not a registered nurse at the time, some people questioned her qualifications to make a tweet about the vaccine. In situations where your qualifications or knowledge are being questioned, Leonie emphasises the importance of using reputable resources to evidence your tweets, such as signposting to the National Institute for Health and Care Excellence or NHS guidance, or resources from the World Health Organization. The evidence is there to back up your knowledge and professional judgement.

Overall, engaging with social media, and Twitter in particular, had lots of benefits for Leonie's learning as a nursing student. It helped her to form her professional identity and share her learning as she progressed through her degree. She also engaged with the NMC code in a practical way, reflecting on how it applied to the situation she was in. Whilst using technology can come with challenges, Leonie's story highlights how you can engage safely and constructively on social media whilst gaining lots of personal and professional benefits.

ADAPTABILITY

Technology is constantly changing, and it can be hard to keep up with. In this chapter, I've tried to deliberately steer away from discussing how to use a specific piece of software or app, as, by the time this chapter is published, it will likely have changed. Right now, whilst I'm writing, Twitter has undergone a change in management, and many users are starting to explore alternative platforms such as Mastodon (2023) or Threads (2023). At the start of the pandemic, very few people had heard of online meeting software like Zoom or Teams; now, most of us have used one or the other. We can't master every piece of technology or predict what will come next; instead, it helps to try and be adaptable and confident when you do use new technology.

The most important bit of advice this chapter will give you when it comes to being digitally literate is to be confident and just try things out. Very little will go wrong if you take some time to look around and explore what something does. If you do make a mistake, then you can use the 'undo' button to reset and try again. Sometimes there will be a tutorial on how to use the app, software or platform, and these can be useful to familiarise yourself with the layout. When engaging with new technology, you will learn more by doing, so don't be afraid to try.

Of course, there will be times when trial and error doesn't work out. You may even be very confident in the platform you are using but want to be able to do something specific or you keep getting an error message. You are unlikely to be the first person to encounter the error or to try to carry out a certain action. I recommend searching for the technology you are trying to use and either the action you are trying to perform or the error message you see. You will likely find some helpful guides that can show you how to make it work. For example, I have been asked how to get page numbering in Word to start on a page other than the first one multiple times, and I can never remember how. Googling 'Word page numbering to start on a specific page' brings up several help pages that show me how to do it.

You do not need to be an expert to be able to get the most out of technology; you just need to be willing to give things a try and search for things if you get stuck.

TIP

If you get stuck with using a new piece of technology, try searching for the problem you've encountered and the name of the software, website or program. Someone else will have had the same issue, and you can usually find a helpful video tutorial or step-by-step guide to follow.

NEXT STEPS

Once you have built your confidence and become comfortable with some of these key areas, why not try sharing them with someone else? Teaching a friend or colleague can be a great way of demonstrating how far your own skills have come whilst sharing something that might help others. It will help cement your learning, as teaching is a skill that often encourages us to be more conscious of our own actions and behaviours. You could volunteer to get involved in one of the many online nursing communities; perhaps you may like to become a volunteer curator for a professional Twitter account like Leonie did.

There are subject-specific tools that can help you navigate your journey as a nursing student. You can find point-of-care apps that can advise you on patient care and management and pharmaceutical apps that you can look up medications on and revision tools for anatomy and physiology. Some will be free, and others may require you to pay. However, it is always worth checking with your university or placement library first, as they may have a subscription you can use. I have avoided making specific recommendations here, as access and cost really do vary widely, so I would talk to other nurses and nursing students about what they are using.

SOCIAL MEDIA

@WeStudentNurse

'#WeWonder How many of you have the BNF App & how often are you using it on placement or as part of your learning?'

@lauraajaynee96

'Downloaded during my first ward placement and use it all the time! Really useful in practice and during assignments and it's a lot quicker and easier than the book, although some wards want you to use the book instead'.

It is useful to check in and think about some of the skills we have discussed within this chapter. With technology evolving all the time and an endless number of new websites or apps appearing, keeping up can seem impossible. Since I have drafted this chapter, artificial intelligence tools like ChatGPT have become well-known, Twitter became X and new social media tools have emerged. However, it is important to remember that technology is only useful if it is useful to you. You might want to go back to the list you made at the start about how you use technology, and think about how this list might have changed and where you might need to improve your skills.

What aspects of your studies, placements or career can technology help you? What would you like to be good at or improve, but have felt nervous to try?

_____

_____

_____

_____

_____

CONCLUSION

There are multiple aspects to digital literacy: information literacy, content creation, communication and collaboration, digital identity and well-being and adaptability. Each component offers a way for you to exploit technology and use it to enhance your learning and career whilst adhering to the NMC code. Understanding how to find and use good-quality information online will ensure you use the best available evidence. Being able to create content digitally will offer you ways to communicate with peers, colleagues and patients through a variety of methods, giving options to improve accessibility. Digital technology allows you to communicate and collaborate across hundreds of miles, saving time from travel but opening your learning up to learn from people outside of your immediate day to day. At the same time, being reflective of your digital identity online will ensure you use social media and other platforms with professionalism whilst setting healthy boundaries to maximise the benefits and protect your own well-being. Last, staying adaptable and thinking creatively about technology will help you continue to develop your skills and overcome any obstacles you encounter.

The future of nursing will require digital capabilities as we find new technological solutions to healthcare. Whilst we cannot know with certainty what they will be, embracing new ideas and staying open to learning will ensure you are ready to meet any new challenges nursing will bring. To stay up to date, it can be useful to connect with relevant online groups or Twitter chats that share their own experiences and can offer tips. You may find that your university, placement area or workplace has a committee or steering group you can be involved with that focuses on digital technology. And of course, your local healthcare library or university librarian will often be able to direct you to resources and sometimes offer training on them. The most important thing is to be open to challenges because there will be lots of opportunities that come with them.

Now you have finished this chapter. Please make notes on what you have learned.

REFERENCES

Bedford, D. (2018) 'Nurses must consider which information to use and trust', *Nursing Times*, 114(9), p. 83.

Canva (2023) *Canva: Free design tool*. Available at: https://www.canva.com/ (Accessed 10 August 2023).

Chartered Institute of Library and Information Professionals (2018) *CILIP definition of information literacy 2018*. Available at: https://infolit.org.uk/ILdefinitionCILIP2018.pdf (Accessed 26 June 2023).

Forest (2023) *Forest – stay focused, be present*. Available at: https://www.forestapp.cc/ (Accessed 10 August 2023)

Health Education England (no date) *What is digital literacy?* Available at: https://digital-transformation.hee.nhs.uk/building-a-digital-workforce/digital-literacy/what-is-digital-literacy (Accessed 26 June 2023).

Health Education England (2018) *A health and care digital capabilities framework*. Available at: https://www.hee.nhs.uk/sites/default/files/documents/Digital%20Literacy%20Capability%20Framework%202018.pdf (Accessed 23 November 2022).

Jisc (2014) *Developing digital literacies*. Available at: https://www.jisc.ac.uk/guides/developing-digital-literacies (Accessed 26 June 2023).

Kahoot (2023) *Kahoot! | Learning games | Make learning awesome!* Available at: https://kahoot.com/ (Accessed 10 August 2023).

Mastodon (2023) *Mastodon – decentralized social media*. Available at: https://join-mastodon.org/ (Accessed 10 August 2023).

Mentimeter (2023) *Interactive presentation software – Mentimeter*. Available at: https://www.mentimeter.com/ (Accessed 10 August 2023).

Miro (2023) *The visual collaboration platform for every team | Miro*. Available at: https://miro.com/ (Accessed 10 August 2023).

Nursing and Midwifery Council (2018) *The code: Professional standards of practice and behaviour for nurses, midwives and nursing associates*. Available at: https://www.nmc.org.uk/globalassets/sitedocuments/nmc-publications/nmc-code.pdf (Accessed 22 November 2022).

Nursing and Midwifery Council (2019) *Social media guidance*. Available at: https://www.nmc.org.uk/standards/guidance/social-media-guidance/ (Accessed 26 June 2023).

Padlet (no date) *Padlet: Beauty will save the work*. Available at: https://padlet.com/ (Accessed 15 August 2023).

Pomofocus (2023) *Time to focus!* Available at: https://pomofocus.io/ (Accessed 10 August 2023).

Quality Watch (2020) *The remote care revolution during Covid-19*. Available at: https://www.nuffieldtrust.org.uk/remote-care-revolution (Accessed 22 November 2022).

The Royal College of Nursing (2018) *Every nurse an e-nurse: Insights from a consultation on the digital future of nursing*. Available at: https://www.rcn.org.uk/Professional-Development/publications/pdf-007013 (Accessed 23 November 2022).

Threads (2023) *Threads*. Available at: https://www.threads.net/ (Accessed 10 August 2023).

Trello (2023) *Manage your team's projects from anywhere | Trello*. Available at: https://trello.com/ (Accessed 15 August 2023).

UNESCO (2023) *Information literacy*. Available at: https://www.unesco.org/en/ifap/information-literacy (Accessed 26 June 2023).

ZoteroBib (2022) *ZoteroBib: Fast, free bibliography generator*. Available at: https://zbib.org/ (Accessed 10 August 2023).

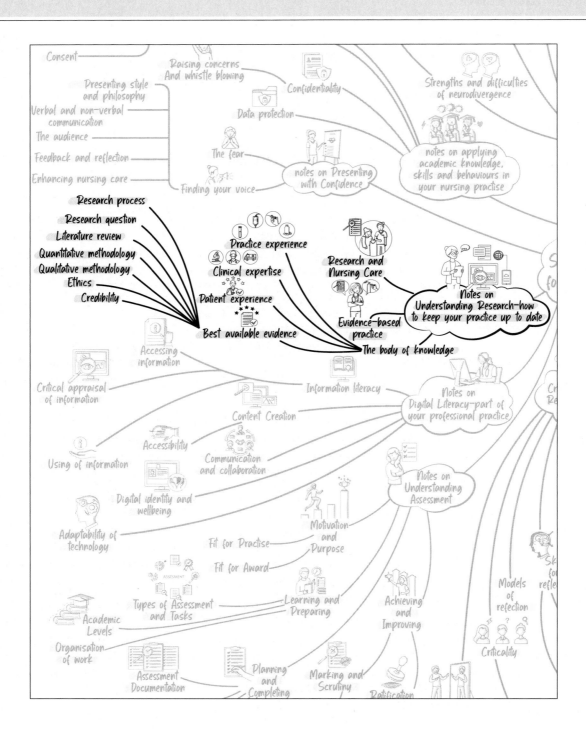

NOTES ON UNDERSTANDING RESEARCH—HOW TO KEEP YOUR PRACTICE UP TO DATE

Dr Julia Williams (she/her)

INTRODUCTION

Nursing research is a powerful tool and plays a crucial role in improving everyday nursing practice. Carrying out research and asking questions about current practice help us learn and update our knowledge to give better care. Many nursing students find the prospect of learning about research daunting and understanding the concept of evidence-based practice overwhelming (Abu-Baker et al., 2021). However, there is a need for all nurses to be able to translate their knowledge and skills to improve patient outcomes and develop professional practice, which will ultimately safeguard the public. Skills in understanding research and the importance of evidence-based practice empower the nurse to do this confidently and competently. This chapter will take you on a journey that encompasses the essence of evidence-based practice. As you delve into the core of this subject, you'll uncover the significance of it as a body of clinical-, patient- and research-based knowledge. You will learn about the research process and the importance of critically appraising and embracing research findings. By honing this knowledge, you're not only enriching your own knowledge but also laying the foundation for a future in nursing practice that is rooted in evidence, ultimately elevating the standard of care provided.

CONNECTING RESEARCH AND NURSING CARE

Research is a core part of the National Health Service (NHS) through its commitment to innovate and promote research activity to improve the current and future health and care of the population. The Care Quality Commission's (2022) appraisal of NHS Hospital Trusts within England found that those trusts associated with research activity clearly contributed to a better patient experience. This suggests that clinical research, the study of health and illness in people, should be seen as more than an academic exercise, as it is a key part of improving patient care.

SOCIAL MEDIA

@RCPhysicians

'Research is a key part of the NHS constitution for England and the benefits it can bring are broad. That's why we are calling for every clinician working in the NHS to be supported to become research active'

Research attempts to gain generalisable new knowledge by addressing clearly defined questions with systematic and rigorous methods. High-quality or best practice can be seen where research findings have been integrated into clinical (medical, nursing, midwifery or allied health professional) decision-making, forming the basis of evidence-based practice. Gerrish and Lathlean (2015, p 4) define research as 'an attempt to increase the sum of what is known, usually referred to as a "body of knowledge" by the discovery of new facts or relationships through a process of systematic scientific enquiry, the research process'.

NMC

THE NMC SAYS

'At the point of registration, the registered nurse will be able to demonstrate an understanding of research methods, ethics and governance in order to critically analyse, safely use, share and apply research findings to promote and inform best nursing practice'.

'Evidence-based person-centred care/nursing care is making sure that any care and treatment is given to people, by looking at what

> research has shown to be most effective. The judgment and experience of the nurse and the views of the person should also be considered when choosing which treatment is most likely to be successful for an individual'.

The values and principles within the Nursing and Midwifery Council (NMC) (2018) code conveys the need to uphold professional knowledge in nursing and midwifery practice in clinical practice, leadership, education and research. 'Practice effectively' indicates that, as nurses, we should always practice aligned to best evidence, making sure that any information or advice given is evidence based. To do this, you need to be research aware, research literate and research confident by developing skills to search for and evaluate evidence to share and apply findings to practice within the context of caring.

NMC

THE NMC SAYS

6.1 'Make sure that any information or advice given is evidence-based including information relating to using any health and care products or services'.

6.2 'Maintain the knowledge and skills you need for safe and effective practice'.

You may have already noted when reading the code (NMC, 2018) that the four core themes stand as guiding principles that connect with research and evidence-based practice. **Prioritise people** echoes the essence of person-centred care, emphasising the integration of research findings into the nursing process. **Practise effectively** underscores the vital role of evidence-based decision-making, where nurses draw from research insights to ensure optimal care. **Preserve safety** resonates with the thorough approach to research methodologies, ensuring rigorousness and ethical considerations. Lastly, **promote professionalism and trust** reflects the imperative for nurses to continuously engage with research to uphold the highest standards of practice, fostering confidence through informed and evidence-driven caregiving. See Table 8.1 for further details.

TABLE 8.1 THE FOUR THEMES OF THE CODE (NMC, 2018) AND EXAMPLES OF HOW THEY ALIGN TO RESEARCH AND EVIDENCE-BASED PRACTICE

Theme	Meaning	Relationship to research and evidence-based practice
Prioritise people	Putting the interests of people using or needing nursing or midwifery services first	• Evaluates evidence • Recognises and understands the needs of people and their families • Regulations
Practise effectively	Assessing need and deliver or advise on treatment, giving help without too much delay, to the best of your abilities, based on best available evidence	• Fosters contemporary practice • Ensures knowledge exchange • Explores the realities of practice • Supports innovation and creativity • Advocates problem-solving and decision-making
Preserve safety	Making sure that patient and public safety are not affected	• Evaluates to improve patient care and safety • Develops policies, procedures and guidelines • Safeguarding the public
Promote professionalism and trust	Upholding the reputation of the profession always	• Builds confidence and knowledge • Develops nursing as a profession • Empowers clinical practice

Source: This extract is reproduced and reprinted with permission with thanks to the Nursing and Midwifery Council. The Code. Professional standards of practice and behaviour for nurses, midwives and nursing associates. London: Nursing and Midwifery Council. 2018.

Why do you do the things you do when on your practice placements?

Can you think of any practices that were previously carried out that would now be considered unhelpful or even harmful?

_____

_____

_____

_____

_____

_____

INTRODUCING EVIDENCE–BASED PRACTICE

What is evidence-based practice?

Evidence-based practice can be defined as the integration of the best research evidence with clinical expertise and the patient's unique values and circumstances (Sackett et al., 2011). Advances in healthcare, such as surgical techniques, drug therapies, diagnostic and therapeutic screening, as well as patient recovery programmes, have contributed to an increased life expectancy and improved disease management for many. For the nurse, and you as a nursing student, there is the constant challenge to keep abreast of these advances and provide more formal, precise and accurate information, facilitating individualised patient need. Aveyard and Sharp (2013, p4) define evidence-based practice as a 'practice supported by a clear, up-to-date rationale, taking into account the patient and/or client's preferences, using the nurse's own judgement as well as best evidential research'.

What counts as evidence and when?

As per the definition by Sackett et al. (2011), and as illustrated in Fig. 8.1, there are three components to evidence-based practice, as it is derived

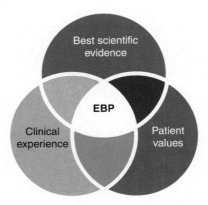

Fig. 8.1   Evidence of best practice (Aveyard and Sharp, 2013). (Source: Summary of Evidence-based Practice (EBP) in Nursing Administration (smu.edu.ph))

from a variety of sources that build a 'body' of knowledge for effective practice.

- *Knowledge from* **clinical expertise/practice experience—**this encompasses the nurse's knowledge, skills and proficiency in their specified area of practice.
- *Knowledge from* **patient experience—preferences and values—** where recognition is made that patients are all individual.
- *Knowledge from* **best available evidence—**this refers to the most current, relevant and reliable research.

Who benefits?

Evidence-based practice undeniably leads to better patient outcomes and enhances safety whilst also empowering nurses to deliver best research-based care.

Benefits to patients

- Promotes positive patient outcomes
- Promotes patient autonomy
- Allows flexibility in care planning

- Prevents and reduces patient complications and unforeseen patient issues

Benefits to nursing

- Helps nurses keep up to date clinically
- Supports the decision-making process
- Develops critical thinking
- Encourages lifelong learning

Benefits to healthcare delivery

- Ensures caregiving is consistent
- Improves patient outcomes
- Ensures resourcing remains efficient
- Supports the delivery of best practice and good-quality care

THE BODY OF KNOWLEDGE FOR EVIDENCE-BASED PRACTICE

Knowledge from practice experience and clinical expertise

What does knowing the patient mean to you?

Think of a scenario where someone has asked you if you know the patient. What did you know, and how did you know?

_____

_____

_____

_____

Nurses play a crucial role in establishing positive and trusting therapeutic relationships with patients, and these are essential for effective care. These relationships are primarily based on mutual trust and also respect, faith, hope and sensitivity to individuals' physical, emotional and spiritual needs (Freshwater, 2007; Mirhaghi et al., 2017). Skills like successful interaction, focusing, knowing, anticipating and evaluating are key for establishing and maintaining these trusting and responsive relationships, ensuring a person-centred approach. The therapeutic relationship begins when you meet the patient, and it requires verbal and nonverbal communication skills, such as senses and physical touch. Emotional intelligence, including self-awareness and empathy, also play a pivotal role in getting to know the people and families you care for.

Nurses also utilise various information sources to support the understanding of patient need and care in acute and community settings. When on placement, you will collect and communicate information through patient records and nursing documentation, ensuring a comprehensive understanding of the person's condition and resulting care plan. In addition, you will use clinical guidelines, 'systematically developed statements to assist practitioner and patient decisions about appropriate healthcare for specific clinical circumstances' (Browman et al., 1995, p 503) to guide you.

The creation of guidelines is promoted and supported by governments and professional organisations as a catalyst for standardising practice so as to provide a benchmark for patient care and treatment. Many countries have established structures at national or regional levels dedicated to compiling evidence and producing guidelines. Additionally, these countries often provide incentives to promote practices aligned with the latest guideline recommendations. In the United Kingdom, we have the National Institute for Health Clinical Excellence (NICE). Using NICE guidance can support and monitor progress or show compliance with national standards, and using NICE quality standards can help demonstrate outstanding performance (NICE, 2023). Peer-reviewed resources are readily available on the website (www.nice.org.uk). Guidelines are an important part of an evidence-based practice toolkit which, transformed into practice recommendations, has the potential to improve both the process of care and patient outcomes.

CASE STUDY

These three studies have demonstrated how practice has improved following the introduction of guidelines. See if you can find them in your library; references are in the list at the end of the chapter.

- In Wakeman et al. (2022)'s study involving paediatric appendectomy cases, the introduction of a clinical practice guideline led to a significant decrease in surgical site infections and overall morbidity. This improvement was achieved by implementing practices such as obtaining intraoperative cultures and administering appropriate antibiotics based on culture data, showcasing how guidelines can enhance patient outcomes and reduce healthcare complications.
- Mowat et al. (2011)'s paper outlines the revision of guidelines, considering critical factors like nationwide audits, service standards, disease classification updates, immunosuppressive therapy and the safe use of biological treatments for better physical functioning outcomes for patients with inflammatory bowel disease.
- In Setkowski et al. (2021)'s study focused on psychiatric care, evidence-based guidelines positively impacted the severity of psychopathological symptoms and reduced the time to remission when compared to treatment as usual. This research underscores the potential of evidence-based guidelines to enhance patient care and emphasises the importance of understanding the mechanisms behind these improvements for routine practice.

Knowledge from patient experience—preferences and values

Personal knowledge and experience of patients and their families and carers present an important source of knowledge, relevant to evidence-based practice. Although subjective, contribution of this knowledge should not be dismissed, and as such, there are two types of evidence available from the patient's perspective: previous experience of care and the patient's own knowledge of themselves (den Hertog and

Niessen, 2019). Review Table 8.2 below, which introduces you to the key skills needed to gather information in relation to assessing the patient for their values and preferences.

Patient, family and carer feedback provides a valuable insight into the care people receive. As nursing students, you'll encounter the gathering and using of patient feedback. It's all about understanding the views and opinions of healthcare experiences. Healthcare organisations employ various methods to collect this, such as surveys, audits and even comments and complaints.

Using feedback gathered and involving people who experience care and use services in decisions about the planning, design and arrangement of

TABLE 8.2 SKILLS NEEDED FOR GATHERING INFORMATION IN RELATION TO ASSESSING THE PATIENT FOR THEIR VALUES AND PREFERENCES	
Need	**Skills**
Get to know your patient	• Introduce yourself and explain your role in the delivery of their care • Refer to #hellomynameis campaign • Utilise documentation, including healthcare records • Observe the patient, both physically and psychologically • Remember this is a continuous process • Demonstrate self- and emotional awareness • Be attentive to every sign or signal from the patient • Transform the information gathered
Gather clues	• Talk to the healthcare team members and observe the patient • Be careful not to make assumptions • Talk to the patient • Observe the patient's actions • Tuning into and picking up on patient cues • Take care not to misinterpret patient's reaction • Read and interrupt the patient's nonverbal cues

TABLE 8.2 SKILLS NEEDED FOR GATHERING INFORMATION IN RELATION TO ASSESSING THE PATIENT FOR THEIR VALUES AND PREFERENCES—cont'd

Need	Skills
Establish a rapport	• Make eye contact when appropriate and help your patient feel comfortable with you • Notice and acknowledge the patient • Actively listen to the patient's thoughts, feelings and concerns (and their families) • Undertake a comprehensive assessment • Recall something the patient has already told you about themselves • Talk to the patient little and often depending on their need • Demonstrate empathy • Evaluate and review progress of the nurse–patient relationship • Remain attentive • Appropriate use of physical touch
Gain trust	• Show respect and treat each patient with compassion • Remain nonjudgemental • Offer explanations using terminology the patient understands • Paraphrase what the patient has told so that you acknowledge what has been said • Be receptive and responsive to patient's nonverbal communication • Display high standard of professional knowledge, self-confidence and concern to gain the patient's trust. Show concern and act as the patient's advocate
Determine your patient's readiness to learn	• Ask your patients about their goals, attitudes and motivations
Learn the patient's perspective	• Talk to the patient about worries, fears and possible misconceptions

Continued

TABLE 8.2 SKILLS NEEDED FOR GATHERING INFORMATION IN RELATION TO ASSESSING THE PATIENT FOR THEIR VALUES AND PREFERENCES—cont'd

Need	Skills
Ask the right questions	• Use open-ended questions that require the patient to reveal more details • Listen carefully • The patient's answers will help you learn their core beliefs
Learn about the patient's skills	• Find out what your patient already knows and build on this knowledge
Involve others	• Identify the significant people in the patient's life • Identify what support they have and what they might need • Collaborate with other healthcare professionals as needed
Good problem-solving skills	• Actively listening • Engage in teamwork • Develop skills in emotional intelligence • Be creative

(Adapted from Williams, 2021, p 50)

care are important to ensure it is relevant and responsive to patient need. In the United Kingdom, there are examples of collective patient involvement in evidence-based practice-related activities (see Table 8.3). The Database of Patients' Experiences (DIPEx) is an example of how patients' experiences can be linked to inform evidence-based practice through research. This work has been ongoing since 2001; further information can be found at https://dipexcharity.org/.

TABLE 8.3 EXAMPLES OF PATIENT-LED CAMPAIGNS

Campaign	Focus	Contact
You can make a difference	Dementia care awareness	https://www.combined.nhs.uk/person-centredness-framework/national-campaigns/you-can-make-difference/
Me Too movement	Sexual harassment and assault reporting	https://metoomvmt.org/
Hello My Name Is	Compassionate care awareness	https://www.hellomynameis.org.uk/
Lives Not Knives	Prevent knife crime	https://www.livesnotknives.org/
Eat Them To Defeat Them	Increasing fruit and vegetable intake in children	https://eatthemtodefeatthem.com/

What different ways, including organisations, services and activities, do you know that facilitate and support people to share their experiences of care in healthcare and NHS organisations?

_____

_____

_____

_____

Knowledge from best available evidence—research-based activity

Research is inclined to take priority over practice experience, clinical expertise and patient preference in relation to evidence-based practice, as there is a perception that it is:

- Robust
- Credible
- Trustworthy

This can only be seen if the researcher has kept in line with the research process. The research process consists of a series of systematic procedures that a researcher must go through in order to generate knowledge that will be considered valuable by the project and focus on the relevant topic (see Fig. 8.2). Once the ideas have been thought through, the research question can be developed.

Developing the research question

Developing a research question can be a difficult and challenging step. It can be defined as a statement of the specific query the researcher wants to answer in order to address the research problem (Polit and Hungler, 2013). In other words, the research question identifies and describes a gap in nursing knowledge, which the researcher seeks to address. Research questions are generated from practical problems in practice, ideas that stem from experience, theories and the literature as well as proposals from funding stakeholders.

The PEO (which stands for Population/patient/problem; Exposure; Outcome) and PICO (which stands for Population/patient/problem; Intervention; Co comparison/context; Outcome) acronyms are used widely in nursing and healthcare research to support the development of research questions. Both the PEO and PICO frameworks have similar elements; the PEO acronym lends itself to qualitative research (see Fig. 8.3 with examples), whilst the PICO lends itself to quantitative research, allowing for comparisons between interventions (see Fig. 8.4 with examples).

Literature review

Literature reviews have grown in importance, as they combine the body of knowledge that is already available, providing an overview. So, a literature review is an objective, thorough summary and critical analysis of the best primary research available on a specific topic (Baker, 2016). Types of literature review include systematic reviews, meta-analyses and meta-synthesis.

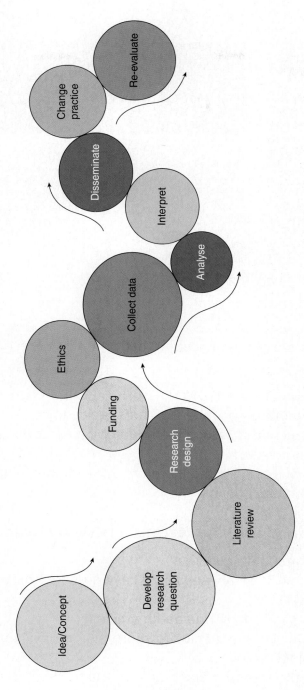

Fig. 8.2 The research process. Summary of Evidence-based Practice (EBP) in Nursing Administration (smu.edu.ph)

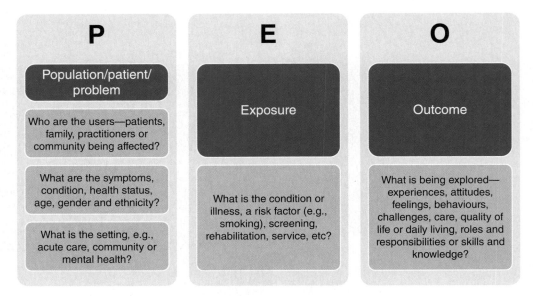

Fig. 8.3   Understanding PEO.

Literature reviews are generally carried out prior to any research activity so as to

- Provide a theoretical framework
- Provide an integrated overview of the specific topic
- Confirm the suitable research methodology and research design for any further research
- Demonstrate any gaps in the literature, for example, what has been done and what hasn't

The process to undertake a literature review includes

- Structuring a research question
- Searching relevant databases using keywords to provide a focus to the search
- Selecting relevant primary research articles
- Critically appraising the articles to score the credibility or trustworthiness of the study
- Synthesising the reported findings from the research articles to determine common themes
- Writing up and sharing

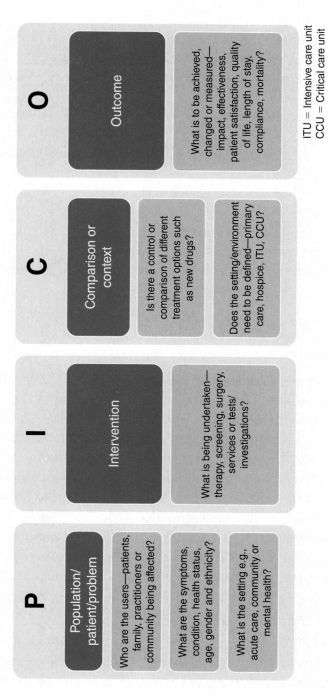

P

Population/
patient/problem

Who are the users—patients, family, practitioners or community being affected?

What are the symptoms, condition, health status, age, gender and ethnicity?

What is the setting e.g., acute care, community or mental health?

I

Intervention

What is being undertaken—therapy, screening, surgery, services or tests/investigations?

C

Comparison or context

Is there a control or comparison of different treatment options such as new drugs?

Does the setting/environment need to be defined—primary care, hospice, ITU, CCU?

O

Outcome

What is to be achieved, changed or measured—impact, effectiveness, patient satisfaction, quality of life, length of stay, compliance, mortality?

ITU = Intensive care unit
CCU = Critical care unit

Fig. 8.4   Understanding PICO.

TIPS FOR DATABASE SEARCHING

- Select a database relevant to your search
- Always carry out an advanced search rather than basic
- Identify keywords for the search, making sure they relate to your question
- Represent each element of your PICO or PEO when selecting keywords
- If searching several databases, always use the same keywords
- Use synonyms
- Make good use of the Boolean operators
- Use truncation
- Apply filters and limits to your search
- Create an account so you can save your search
- Remember, searching can be laborious, so stagger the time spent searching

Research design

When planning any research activity, there is a need to identify which methodology will be selected to best answer the research question, for example, quantitative or qualitative methodologies (Ellis, 2022). More recently, studies have been seen to use a blend of both methodologies, as they both seem to contribute to the overall findings of a study. This type of study is referred to as mixed methodology, as it combines quantitative and qualitative data collection and analysis. Individually, these approaches can answer different questions, so combining them can provide more in-depth findings (Creswell, 2014). For example, a new drug therapy might have been tested, using a quantitative method, reporting very good treatment outcomes. Using qualitative data in the same study would offer the experiences of the patient taking the new drug to explore if there are any changes in lifestyle that have been imposed by the new treatment that might cause concern.

There are many terms used within research; some are general terms, and others are more specific to the type of methodology. Table 8.4 outlines some that relate to both qualitative and quantitative research.

TABLE 8.4 GENERAL RESEARCH TERMINOLOGY

Research term	Meaning
Data	Information collected from participants to be analysed later
Methodology	Are the plans and procedures that span the steps from broad assumptions to detailed methods of data collection, analysis and interpretation, referred to as quantitative or qualitative methodologies
Paradigm	The particular way of viewing a phenomenon in the world, worldview
Participant	Individual recruited to take part in the study
Primary research	Studies that are first hand narratives, original studies, factual accounts
Research design	Types of inquiry that provide specific direction for procedures in a study
Research method	Involves the forms, types of data collection, analysis and interpretation
Sampling	The process of selecting participants for the study. The sample is chosen from the total possible data sources, namely, the population
Secondary research	Studies that interpret, analyse and critique primary sources, providing a second-hand version of events, such as literature reviews

Familiarising yourself with these terms and unpicking the definitions will enable a better comprehension of research studies.

Quantitative methodology

Quantitative methodologies tend to follow a scientific method, emphasising objectively by seeking to remove bias at each point of the research process. Taking a positivist perspective, the researcher is seen as an impartial observer whose role is to infer laws that explain relationships between observed phenomena (Giddens, 2006). Quantitative research methods veer towards measurements and quantity, which are analysed using statistics to establish relationships between variables.

Quantitative methods would be used to test a hypothesis which, through statistical testing, would recognise differences and correlations (Parahoo, 2014). As a result, quantitative studies generate larger sample sizes (Creswell, 2014), so they can conduct meaningful tests on their statistics. This can lead to sampling issues because of the need to be able to create statistical generalisations that are applicable to the wider population (Williamson and Whittaker, 2020).

Quantitative methods offer the opportunity to use different designs to carry out experiments, such as

- Randomised control trials
- Quasi- and nonquasiexperiments
- Surveys

Data are collected via validated or nonvalidated questionnaires and/or measurements, for example, height, weight, blood pressure and urinalysis.

Quantitative analysis

As quantitative research is based on objective measurement, observation as well as concern with correlation and causation, quantitative analysis is a technique that uses mathematical and statistical modelling, measurement and research to understand patterns. Quantitative researchers represent a given reality in terms of a numerical value. Such data may involve descriptive or inferential statistics (Polit and Hungler, 2013). Descriptive statistics describe and synthesise data and show patterns and trends (Burns and Grove, 2009), whereas inferential statistics permit the researcher to infer whether relationships noted in a sample might occur in a larger population (Polit and Hungler, 2013). To determine a significant result, the statistics must have levels of significance. Quantitative data analysis is supported by software packages such as Statistical Package for the Social Sciences (SPSS) (IBM, 2023).

Research terminology relating to quantitative research methods is quite different to those relating to qualitative terms. As you build your confidence with research, you are likely to find you have a preference for one methodology or the other, so familiarising yourself with the differences is important. Table 8.5 can be used as a guide to support this familiarisation.

TABLE 8.5 QUANTITATIVE RESEARCH TERMINOLOGY

Term	Meaning
Bias	Occurs if the researcher's beliefs or expectations influence the research design or data collection
Chi-square	Statistical measurement
CI	Whenever a mean is calculated using a sample, there is always the possibility of error, so the CI is calculated to represent how true the estimate is
Correlation	A mutual relationship or connection between two or more things
Causation	The relationship between cause and effect between one event or action and the result
Hypothesis	A proposed explanation made on the basis of limited information at the starting point of the investigation
Mean	Average score or value
Median	Exact middle score or value
Mode	The value that occurs most frequently in a distribution of scores
Pilot study	A trial run of the research
Positivist	Has an objective perspective
Probability	Likelihood of a particular outcome
p-value	Statistical measurement for probability
Quasiexperiment	Experiment undertaken when the investigation variables cannot clearly be controlled or blinded
RCT	Experiment where participants are randomly assigned to one of two groups: experimental and control. Referred to as the 'gold standard' in healthcare research
Random sampling	Probability sampling method

Continued

TABLE 8.5 QUANTITATIVE RESEARCH TERMINOLOGY—cont'd

Term	Meaning
Statistic	Involves the collection, description, analysis and inference of conclusions from quantitative data
Significance	A quality of being worthy of attention
SPSS	Statistical Package for the Social Sciences
Standard deviation	The spread of data from the mean value
Survey	A descriptive snapshot of the current situation

CI, Confidence interval; *RCT*, randomised control trial.

Qualitative methodology

Qualitative methodologies take an interpretivist approach to understand the world from various perspectives and are therefore viewed as subjective (Holloway and Galvin, 2017). Qualitative research takes an interest in people's lived experience and the progressive nature of the experience.

Qualitative methods are concerned with the true-to-life description or interpretation of experiences in terms of the meanings these have for the people experiencing them. This contrasts with quantitative methods, which are concerned with counting the amount of phenomenon or some aspect concerning this. The inductive and flexible nature of qualitative data collection methods offers unique advantages in relation to quantitative inquiry (Holloway and Galvin, 2017). The biggest advantage is the ability to probe into responses or observations as needed and obtain more detailed descriptions and explanations of experiences, behaviours and beliefs.

Qualitative research may seem intuitive and subjective (Holloway and Galvin, 2017); however, as critics of evidence-based practice are quick to point out, clinical practice itself is more than the application of systematic rules. It has long been criticised for being merely a collection of anecdotal and personal impressions, leading to its subjectivity to be seen as a poor basis for making scientific decisions (Speziale and

Carpenter, 2011). Holloway and Galvin (2017) point out that clinical expe-rience, based on personal observation, reflection and judgement, is also needed to translate scientific outcome into treatment of individual patients. Therefore, qualitative research aligns with the nursing thera-peutic philosophy (Leininger, 1985) for empathising a holistic under-standing of the subject matter (Gray and Grove, 2020). All qualitative research links people's subjective experiences, perceptions, thoughts and feelings and lived phenomena; it explores the whole phenomena revealed in and through individuals (Crotty, 1996).

Approaches to qualitative research include:

- Grounded theory
- Ethnography
- Phenomenology (descriptive and interpretive)
- Case studies

In contrast to quantitative methods, qualitative studies aim to generate extensive data with the smaller samples that they are researching; therefore, participants are selected purposively. This is commonly used in qualitative research for the identification and selection of information-rich cases related to the phenomenon of interest. Methods of data col-lection allow participants to offer 'a rich, detailed, first-person account of their experiences' (Smith et al., 2009, p 56) and advocate observa-tion, in-depth interviews and focus groups. For most approaches, data are collected until the point of data saturation has been reached.

Qualitative analysis

In qualitative research, the process by which data analysis is undertaken is fundamental to determining the credibility of the findings. Essentially, analysis allows the transformation of the data collected so that the nar-rative from the participants can be translated into themes (Speziale and Carpenter, 2011).

Thematic analysis is referred to as a method for identifying, analysing and reporting patterns (themes) within the data (Braun and Clarke, 2021). Smith et al (2009) describes thematic analysis as an iterative and inductive cycle which proceeds to draw upon the following: close line-by-line analysis of the claims, concerns and understandings of each participant; identification of emerging patterns, coding data and developing relationships with data relative to context; organisation of data for purposes of audit trail; develop coherence and plausibility of interpretation and, finally, personal reflection.

As previously mentioned, having familiarisation with research terminology eases your understanding of research and therefore supports research awareness. Table 8.6 provides an overview of terms associated with qualitative research.

TABLE 8.6 QUALITATIVE RESEARCH TERMINOLOGY	
Term	**Meaning**
Case studies	Explores the development of a particular person, group or situation over time
Data saturation	The point in the research process when no new information is disclosed when collecting data
Deductive	Draws conclusions from patterns
Ethnography	Explores the behaviours, thoughts and attitudes of cultural groups
Focus groups	Group interview
Grounded theory	Generates theory directly from the data
Hawthorn effect	Occurs when people behave differently because they know they are being watched
Inductive	Draws conclusions from what has been observed
Interpretivist	Has a subjective perspective
Interviews	Conversation where the researcher asks the participant questions in relation to the topic being explored: structured, semistructured and unstructured
Observation	Process of watching the participant(s) closely as a participant or nonparticipant
Phenomenology	In-depth focus—human experiences as they are lived
Purposive sampling	Nonprobability sample that is selected by characteristics of the population

TIPS TO IDENTIFY PRIMARY RESEARCH ARTICLES

- Almost always published in a peer-reviewed journal
- Asks a research question or states a hypothesis
- Identifies the research population
- Describes a specific research method
- Will explore, measure or test something
- States the method of data collection (questionnaire, interview, focus group, observations)
- Indicates how the participants were sampled for the study
- Confirms ethical approval has been sought and achieved
- Seen to undertake an analysis of the data collected
- Presents the findings as statistics or participants narratives
- Draws upon conclusions
- Considers implications of practice
- Declares any conflicts of interest

Ethics

All those involved in healthcare research need to have an awareness of their ethical and legal duty to protect the participants during the process of carrying it out. Ethical principles are universal and should be upheld whether conducting research, audit or service evaluation. The NMC (2018) code contains a series of statements that, taken together, signify what good practice by nurses, midwives and nursing associates looks like. It puts the interests of patients and service users first, is safe and effective and promotes trust through professionalism.

NMC

THE NMC SAYS

5.2 'Make sure that people are informed about how and why information is used and shared by those who will be providing care'.

10.6 'Collect, treat and store all data and research findings appropriately'.

17.1 'Take all reasonable steps to protect people who are vulnerable or at risk from harm, neglect or abuse'.

Continued

17.2 'Share information if you believe someone may be at risk of harm, in line with the laws relating to the disclosure of information'.

19.1 'Take measures to reduce as far as possible, the likelihood of mistakes, near misses, harm and the effect of harm if it takes place'.

20.2 'Act with honesty and integrity at all times, treating people fairly and without discrimination, bullying or harassment'.

21.3 'Act with honesty and integrity'.

21.4 'Make sure that any advertisements, publications or published material you produce or have produced for your professional services are accurate, responsible, ethical, do not mislead or exploit vulnerabilities and accurately reflect your relevant skills, experience and qualifications'.

21.6 'Cooperate with the media only when it is appropriate to do so, and then always protecting the confidentiality and dignity of people receiving treatment or care'.

The NMC (2018) code serves as a key guide, with consideration of the core ethical principles of nonmaleficence, beneficence, autonomy and justice. Table 8.7 illustrates these principles. Clearly, research participants have inherent rights that allow them to make informed decisions about taking part in a study as well as withdrawing from it. Researchers must instil confidence in the participant, allowing them to make informed decisions about participating in a study, and during and after participation, to be treated in a safe, humane and professional manner.

Ethics approval panels set out to monitor research activity. The panels generally meet monthly, consisting of healthcare professionals and people who receive care and/or use services, often referred to as experts by experience.

Service evaluation and audit

Knowing the difference between research and service evaluation or audit can be difficult to determine. The purpose of each is to contribute

TABLE 8.7 KEY ETHICAL PRINCIPLES RELATED TO RESEARCH

Key principle	Meaning	Considerations
Beneficence	Try to do good	Who will benefit and in what way? • Research participants—in what way? • Future patients/clients/services? • Is a body of knowledge likely to be increased? • Will the researcher gain educationally from conducting the study? • If there is no benefit for anyone, is the study ethical? • Identify anticipated benefits when justifying research.
Nonmalevolence	Do no harm	Are the participants protected and come to no harm? • Consider the possibility of physical and/or psychological harm • Justify procedures • Weigh up risks versus benefits • Not all participants require the same degree of 'protection' • Once identified, mitigate risks
Respect for autonomy	Transparency	Is there autonomy which acknowledges people can determine their own goals and needs • Full information is required to make autonomous decisions • Consent is an expression of autonomy • Privacy and confidentiality are obligations under this principle

Continued

TABLE 8.7 KEY ETHICAL PRINCIPLES RELATED TO RESEARCH—cont'd

Key principle	Meaning	Considerations
Informed consent	Permission given/received in full knowledge of the possible outcomes	Has the participant been provided with enough information to understand the research activity and make an informed choice to be part of the study? • Seek informed consent in writing • Information—amount, level and how it is communicated • Use simple language (aim for the reading age of 12 years old) • Decision—conscious process to consent or to refuse, not to just accept • Voluntariness—freedom from coercion • Requires full information, clearly communicated • Risks and benefits (if any) must be explained
Confidentiality and/or Anonymity	Confidentiality—removing or modifying or personal or identifiable information Anonymity—not obtaining it	Researchers have an obligation to protect identities and locations in storage, access to and reporting of research • Research must not infringe an individual's right to privacy • No public disclosure that identifies individuals (unless court subpoena) • Data should be stored securely and be password protected • Data should be coded • No access to individual records unless expressed consent from participant

TABLE 8.7 KEY ETHICAL PRINCIPLES RELATED TO RESEARCH—cont'd

Key principle	Meaning	Considerations
Justice	Being impartial reasonable and equitable	**Justice** • Acts as safeguard for participants and researchers • Required by law for some studies • Requirement of many professional bodies/funding agencies **Fair play** • Information must be accurate and realistic • Participants can decline to be involved or withdraw without giving a reason • Equal treatment of participants • Prevention of discrimination
Integrity	Being honest and fair	**Integrity** • Treating others the way you want to be treated yourself • Thinking of others before themselves • Treating patients with respect • Offer the same level of care to all regardless of culture, religion or educational background

to what is already known about a certain topic and thus inform, guide and advise best practice.

- **Service evaluations** seek to assess how well a service is achieving its intended aim. It is undertaken to improve service provision, redefining it as needed.
- **Audit** involves quality improvement by measuring existing practice against a predetermined standard.

Some of the evaluation process overlaps research, for example, data collection and analysis. In some healthcare and NHS organisations, ethical approval is required, whilst other areas require approval from clinical governance, which is the department responsible for maintaining and improving care quality. However, ethical principles are universal and should be upheld whether conducting research, audit or service evaluation.

Gathering credible literature

Whilst research plays an important factor in supporting the decision-making process without acknowledging the credibility of the research, the question of whether the findings can be trusted or, indeed, how they were obtained needs to be addressed. Often, the media portrays a news story that makes unjustified healthcare claims; the recent COVID-19 outbreak is an example of this, where, as a result, news events released by the media caused more panic among the public such as number of variants of the disease, poor food supplies and poor distribution of PPE for healthcare workers. More recently, the media has focused on long COVID and how those affected are likely to face unfair treatment (Stewart, 2023), based on evidence from a trade union and charity supporting people with COVID. For those in the know, it is easy to question such reporting, but there is still the risk of sending out incorrect and inappropriate messages unless we can be certain what is being reported is credible.

CASE STUDY

One of the most famous (and serious) cases of research fraud in recent years is that of Andrew Wakefield (Rao and Andrade, 2011). In 1998, Andrew Wakefield and 12 of his colleagues published a case series in the *Lancet* (Wakefield et al., 1998), which suggested that the measles, mumps and rubella (MMR) vaccine may predispose to behavioural regression and pervasive developmental disorder in children. Despite the small sample size ($n = 12$), the uncontrolled design and the speculative nature of the conclusions, the paper received wide publicity, and MMR vaccination rates began to drop because parents were concerned about the risk of autism after vaccination.

CASE STUDY—cont'd

Further studies (Taylor et al., 1999; Dales et al., 2001) ensued refuting the reported outcomes of the origin study with a result of the *Lancet* retracting the Wakefield (1998) paper and a legal battle whereby Andrew Wakefield was removed from the GMC register, resulting in him not being able to practice as a doctor in the United Kingdom (record of licensed doctors in the UK). Although a unique case, this scenario demonstrates the importance of not accepting research as being 100% truth; therefore, the recommendation to critically appraise research prior to implementation is vital.

See if you can find the Wakefield et al. (1998) article in your library or via an online search; the full reference is in the list at the end of the chapter. Once accessed, note how it is labelled retracted throughout.

Critical appraisal and hierarchy of evidence

To achieve confidence in evidence-based practice, nurses must verify that the information is valid, reliable and applicable. Two ways to determine this are critical appraisal and hierarchy of evidence.

Critical appraisal. Poorly conducted research seriously compromises the integrity of the research process; therefore, critical appraisal of its quality is central to inform healthcare decision-making. Critical appraisal is the process of carefully and systematically examining research evidence to judge its trustworthiness, its value and relevance in a particular context (Caldwell et al., 2011). It allows you to use research evidence reliably and efficiently. Critical appraisal skills develop overtime and are intended to enhance expertise in determining whether the research evidence is true and relevant to patients. You can best explain the reasoning for your decisions and actions when you understand the worth of the research supporting practice.

TIPS OF WHERE YOU CAN FIND GOOD CRITICAL APPRAISAL INFORMATION, RESOURCES AND TOOLS

- **JBI** (formerly known as Joanna Briggs Institute)—https://jbi.global/
- **CASP** (Critical Appraisal Skills Programme)—https://casp-uk.net/
- **CEBM** (The Centre for Evidence-Based Medicine)—https://www.cebm.net/

Articles (full references in the reference list)

- Framework for critiquing health research by Caldwell, Henshaw and Taylor (2011)
- How to appraise quantitative research by Cathala and Moorley (2018)
- How to appraise mixed methods research by Moorley and Cathala (2019a)
- How to appraise qualitative research by Moorley and Cathala (2019b)

TIPS FOR CRITICAL APPRAISAL—ASK THE FOLLOWING QUESTIONS:

- What is the aim of the research?
- Is the research methodology appropriate?
- How did the researchers collect the data?
- How was the data analysed?
- Are the results clearly presented?

Hierarchy of evidence. There is a requirement to seek the best available evidence, and in order to understand this, knowledge of the hierarchy of evidence is required. Fig. 8.5 illustrates how the hierarchy of evidence refers to a ranking system whereby a range of different methodologies are graded according to the validity of their findings (Evans, 2003).

Several hierarchies of evidence have been developed to enable different research methods to be ranked according to the validity of their findings. However, most have focused on evaluation of the effectiveness of interventions (Gray and Grove, 2020). Whilst these levels are an important element of evidence-based practice, this chapter has already alluded to research not being perfect. In saying that, understanding these levels

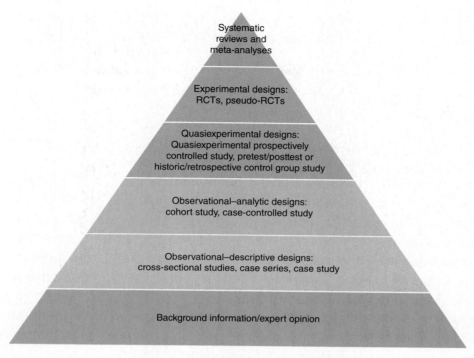

Fig. 8.5 **Hierarchy of evidence.**

and why different methods of information gathering have been assigned to them helps with the prioritising of information. However, it is important to consider all levels and give caution to how outcomes are interpreted.

 TIPS TO ENSURING YOUR PRACTICE IS EVIDENCE-BASED

- **Ask lots of questions**
- **Be curious to seek to understand the 'how' and 'why'**
- **Know your patient**
- **Keep yourself updated**
- **Search health-related databases for journals with peer-reviewed articles that relate to your area of interest**
- **Draw upon your practice placement experiences**
- **Critically evaluate and appraise the research studies you find**
- **Integrate this evidence with what you know and the patient's preferences**
- **Continuously monitor and evaluate the outcome**

Be aware that not all evidence is equal, which means you should look to high-quality, peer-reviewed research when making evidence-based decisions.

CONCLUSION

This chapter has explored evidence-based practice in nursing and why it's so crucial for delivering high-quality patient outcomes. You discovered the multifaceted nature of the evidence base and learned to recognise the diverse sources of knowledge, including 'practice experience', 'clinical expertise' and the invaluable insights from 'patient experience'. Primarily, this chapter has helped you acquire and develop the knowledge, skills and strategies to understand research, the 'best available evidence', taking you through key aspects of the research process. We delved into crafting the right research questions, conducting literature reviews and mastering the art of research design, both quantitative and qualitative. We embraced ethics as the compass guiding our research endeavours and explored the practical aspects of service evaluation and audit. Throughout this chapter, we've uncovered the essence of gathering credible literature and honed our skills in critical appraisal and understanding of the hierarchy of evidence. Evidence-based practice is not a destination; it's an ongoing commitment to delivering the best care to people. The need to adapt to a critical appraisal approach to your reading of research will support the development of future nursing practice. As we move towards an age of digital healthcare, we mustn't lose the fundamentals of nursing, ensuring the care we deliver is of a high standard. Keep your curiosity alive, your critical thinking sharp and your commitment to evidence-based practice unwavering. You are the future of healthcare, and your journey has just begun.

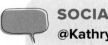

SOCIAL MEDIA
@KathrynFairbro2

'Research is tomorrows care today'

Now you have finished this chapter. Please make notes on what you have learned.

_____

_____

_____

_____

_____

_____

_____

_____

_____

_____

_____

_____

_____

_____

_____

_____

_____

_____

_____

REFERENCES

Abu-Baker, N.N., AbuAlrub, S., Obeidat, R.F. and Assmairan, K. (2021) 'Evidence-based practice beliefs and implementations: a cross-sectional study among undergraduate nursing students', *BMC Nursing*, 20(1), p. 13. Available at: https://doi.org/10.1186/s12912-020-00522-x.

Aveyard, H. and Sharp, P. (2013) *A Beginner's Guide to Evidence-Based Practice in Health and Social Care.* Maidenhead: McGraw Hill.

Baker, J.D. (2016) 'The purpose, process, and methods of writing a literature review', *AORN Journal*, 103(3), pp. 265–269. Available at: https://doi.org/10.1016/j.aorn.2016.01.016.

Browman, G.P., Levine, M.N., Mohide, E.A., Hayward, R.S., Pritchard, K.I., Gafni, A. and Laupacis, A. (1995) 'The practice guidelines development cycle: a conceptual tool for practice guidelines development and implementation', *Journal of Clinical Oncology: Official Journal of the American Society of Clinical Oncology*, 13(2), pp. 502–512. Available at: https://doi.org/10.1200/JCO.1995.13.2.502.

Braun, V., and Clarke, V. (2021) *Thematic Analysis.* London: Sage Publications.

Burns, N. and Grove, S.K. (2003) *The Practice of Nursing Research: Conduct, Critique and Utilization.* 3rd ed. Philadelphia: W.B Saunders.

Burns, N. and Grove, S.K. (2009) *The Practice of Nursing Research. Appraisal, Synthesis, and Generation of Evidence.* 6th ed. Philadelphia: W.B Saunders.

Caldwell, K., Henshaw, L. and Taylor, G. (2011) 'Developing a framework for critiquing health research: an early evaluation', *Nurse Education Today*, 31(8), pp. e1–e7. Available at: https://doi.org/10.1016/j.nedt.2010.11.025.

Cathala, X. and Moorley, C. (2018) 'How to appraise quantitative research', *Evidence-Based Nursing*, 21(4), pp. 99–101. Available at: https://doi.org/10.1136/eb-2018-102996.

Care Quality Commission (2022) *State of care 2021/22 - Care Quality Commission.* Available at: https://www.cqc.org.uk/publication/state-care-202122 (Accessed 3 September 2023).

Creswell, J.W. (2014) *Research Design: Qualitative, Quantitative and Mixed Method Approaches.* 4th Ed. Thousand Oaks: Sage.

Crotty, M. (1998). *The Foundations of Social Research: Meaning and Perspective in the Research Process.* London: SAGE Publications Inc

Dales, L., Hammer, S.J. and Smith, N.J. (2001) 'Time trends in autism and in MMR immunization coverage in California', *Journal of the American Medical Association*, 285(9), pp. 1183–1185. Available at: https://doi.org/10.1001/jama.285.9.1183.

Ellis, P. (2022) *Understanding Research for Nursing Students.* 5th ed. Exeter: Learning Matters Ltd.

Evans, D. (2003) 'Hierarchy of evidence: a framework for ranking evidence evaluating healthcare interventions', *Journal of Clinical Nursing*, 12(1), pp. 77–84. Available at: https://doi.org/10.1046/j.1365-2702.2003.00662.x.

Freshwater, D. (2007) The therapeutic use of self. In: Freshwater, D, (Ed), *Therapeutic Nursing: Improving Patient Care Through Self-Awareness and Reflection.* Sage, London.

Gerrish, K. and Lathlean, J. (2015) *The Research Process in Nursing.* Chichester: John Wiley & Sons.

Giddens, A. (2006) *Sociology.* 5th ed. Cambridge: Polity Press.

Gray, J.R. and Grove, S.K. (2020) *Burn and Grove's the practice of nursing research: appraisal, synthesis and generation of evidence.* 9th ed. Elsevier, Oxford

den Hertog, R. and Niessen, T. (2019) The role of patient preferences in nursing decision-making in evidence-based practice: excellent nurses communication tools. *Journal of Advanced Nursing.* 75(9), 1987–1995 https://doi.org/10.1111/jan.14083

Holloway, I. and Galvin, K. (2017) *Qualitative Research in Nursing and Healthcare.* 4th ed. Chichester: John Wiley & Sons Inc.

IBM (2023) *SPSS Statistics.* Available at: https://www.ibm.com/products/spss-statistics (Accessed 3 September 2023).

Leininger, M.M. (1985) *Qualitative Research Methods in Nursing.* Ed. London, Grune and Stratton

Mirhaghi, A., Sharafi, S., Bazzi, A. and Hasanzadeh, F. (2017) Therapeutic relationship: Is it still heart of nursing? *Nursing Reports.* 7(1). Available at: https://doi.org/10.4081/nursep.2017.6129

Moorley, C. and Cathala, X. (2019a) 'How to appraise mixed methods research', *Evidence-Based Nursing,* 22(2), pp. 38–41. Available at: https://doi.org/10.1136/ebnurs-2019-103076.

Moorley, C. and Cathala, X. (2019b) 'How to appraise qualitative research', *Evidence-Based Nursing,* 22(1), pp. 10–13. Available at: https://doi.org/10.1136/ebnurs-2018-103044.

Mowat, C., Cole, A., Windsor, A., Ahmad, T., Arnott, I., Driscoll, R., Mitton, S., Orchard, T., Rutter, M., Younge, L., Lees, C., Ho, G., Satsangi, J. and Bloom, S. (2011) 'Guidelines for the management of inflammatory bowel disease in adults', *Gut,* 60(5), pp. 571–607. Available at: https://doi.org/10.1136/gut.2010.224154.

National Institute for Health and Care Excellence (2023) *NICE | The National Institute for Health and Care Excellence, NICE.* NICE. Available at: https://www.nice.org.uk/ (Accessed 3 September 2023).

Nursing and Midwifery Council (2018) *The code. Professional standards of practice and behaviour for nurses, midwives and nursing associates.* London: Nursing and Midwifery Council. Available at: https://www.nmc.org.uk/globalassets/sitedocuments/nmc-publications/nmc-code.pdf (Accessed 3 October 2022).

Parahoo, K. (2014) *Nursing Research: Principles, Process and Issues.* Basingstoke: Palgrave MacMillan.

Polit, D.F. and Hungler, B.P. (2013) *Essentials of Nursing Research: Methods, Appraisal, and Utilization.* 8th ed. Philadelphia: Wolters Kluwer/Lippincott Williams and Wilkins.

Sackett, D.L., Strauss, S.E., Richardson, W.S., Rosenberg, W., and Haynes, R.B. (2011) *Evidence Based Medicine: How To Practice and Teach it.* 4th ed., London: Churchill Livingstone.

Rao, T.S.S. and Andrade, C. (2011) 'The MMR vaccine and autism: sensation, refutation, retraction, and fraud', *Indian Journal of Psychiatry,* 53(2), p. 95. Available at: https://doi.org/10.4103/0019-5545.82529.

Setkowski, K., Boogert, K., Hoogendoorn, A.W., Gilissen, R. and van Balkom, A.J.L.M. (2021) 'Guidelines improve patient outcomes in specialised mental health care: a systematic review and meta-analysis', *Acta Psychiatrica Scandinavica,* 144(3), pp. 246–258. Available at: https://doi.org/10.1111/acps.13332.

Smith, J., Flowers, P., and Larkin, M. (2009). *Interpretative Phenomenological Analysis: Theory, Method and Research*. Sage Publications.

Stewart, H. (2023) 'Two-thirds of UK workers with long Covid have faced unfair treatment, says report', *The Guardian*, 26 March. Available at: https://www.theguardian.com/society/2023/mar/27/long-covid-two-thirds-workers-unfair-treatment-report (Accessed 3 March 2023).

Speziale, H.S. and Carpenter, D.R. (2011) *Qualitative Research in Nursing: Advancing the Humanistic Imperative*. 5th ed. Philadelphia: Wolters Kluwer Health/Lippincott Williams & Wilkins.

Taylor, B., Miller, E., Farrington, C.P., Petropoulos, M.C., Favot-Mayaud, I., Li, J. and Waight, P.A. (1999) 'Autism and measles, mumps, and rubella vaccine: no epidemiological evidence for a causal association', *Lancet*, 353(9169), pp. 2026–2029. Available at: https://doi.org/10.1016/s0140-6736(99)01239-8.

Wakefield, A.J., Murch, S.H., Anthony, A., Linnell, J., Casson, D.M., Malik, M., Berelowitz, M., Dhillon, A.P., Thomson, M.A., Harvey, P., Valentine, A., Davies, S.E. and Walker-Smith, J.A. (1998) 'Ileal-lymphoid-nodular hyperplasia, non-specific colitis, and pervasive developmental disorder in children', *Lancet (London, England)*, 351(9103), pp. 637–641. Available at: https://doi.org/10.1016/s0140-6736(97)11096-0.

Wakeman, D., Livingston, M.H., Levatino, E., Juviler, P., Gleason, C., and Tesini B. (2022) 'Reduction of surgical site infections in paediatric patients with complicated appendicitis: Utilization of antibiotic stewardship principles and quality improvement methodology'. *Journal of Paediatric Surgery*, 57(1), pp. 63–73 Available at: https://doi.org/10.1016/j.jpedsurg.2021.09.031.

Williams, J. (2021) 'Information gathering'. In Peate, I. ed *The Nursing Associates Handbook of Clinical Skills*. Ch 6, 44–52. Oxford: Wiley-Blackwell.

Williamson, G.R., and Whittaker, A. (2020) *Succeeding in Literature Reviews and Research Project Plans for Nursing Students*. 4th ed. London: Transforming Nursing Practice series. Sage.

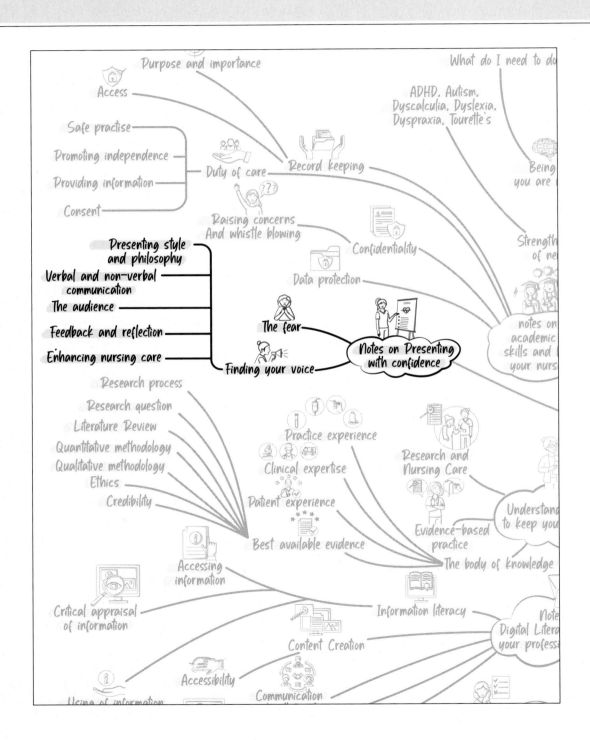

NOTES ON PRESENTING WITH CONFIDENCE

Charlotte Jakab-Hall (she/her)

INTRODUCTION

Welcome to the captivating world of presenting and public speaking! In this chapter, unlock your inner charisma and transform into a captivating speaker. Say goodbye to nervous jitters and hello to unshakeable confidence. Discover your unique speaking philosophy and unleash your authentic voice, setting yourself apart as a nurse with a powerful message. This chapter is designed to enhance your skills, from boosting spontaneity to honing your storytelling prowess. Get ready to command the stage, leaving your audience immersed and inspired. It's time to let your inner voice soar and share your invaluable ideas with the world.

The real fear behind presenting

This chapter could easily reel off how to put together a great presentation, but the truth is that the building of a presentation is just one aspect of presenting with confidence. Not to mention that there are hundreds, if not thousands, of resources online with regards to setting up a good presentation, and of course, delivering a presentation is only one way you will present information as a nursing student or registered nurse. Evidence suggests that the most challenging aspect of any presenting is the public speaking part (Grieve et al., 2021). Picture this: you're standing in front of a group of people, preparing to speak, and suddenly, you find yourself in a state of disarray and at a standstill. You can no longer seem to find the words, your heart rate elevates and your mouth becomes drier than the Sahara desert. Does this feel familiar? Or perhaps you find yourself unintentionally trying to make the Guinness World Record for most words spoken in a 10-minute presentation, struggling to be articulate and reflect the eloquence you practiced or have inside your brilliant mind. Well then, join the club; in fact, glossophobia, or 'the fear of public speaking', as it is better known, is actually a very common phobia to have. It is believed to affect over 75% of the global population (Black, 2019). In fact, it is even suggested that most of the human race hates public speaking so much that they would rather die than give a presentation or speak in public to a crowd (Furmark et al., 1999).

Phew! You're not alone, and the good news is that while the fear of public speaking is common, it is also a skill set that can be taught and learnt. The big question remains: why should I take action to overcome this common fear? Well, it's important to build self-confidence in presenting information because this will follow you throughout your career; whether it's presenting coursework, at an interview for a job, handing over on shift, advocating for your patients and colleagues or simply talking with patients and relatives, public speaking is core to nursing care delivery.

SOCIAL MEDIA
@rachelcannnn

'Being able to speak in public is a taught skill in itself. Having the ability gives nurses confidence to speak up to advocate for patients and themselves more effectively. it's a desirable skill to have but the benefits of it can really help nurses throughout their career'.

Public speaking is a form of communication, and the Nursing and Midwifery Council (NMC) (2018) code clearly identifies that nurses are required to deliver a range of clear, effective, verbal and nonverbal communication methods as a core part of their practice.

NMC

THE NMC SAYS

7.1 'Use terms that people in your care, colleagues and the public can understand'.

7.3 'Use a range of verbal and non-verbal communication methods, and consider cultural sensitivities, to better understand and respond to people's personal and health needs.

7.5 'Be able to communicate clearly and effectively in English'.

Finding your voice in the classroom and beyond

Embrace the reality that public speaking will be a constant companion on your nursing journey. By acknowledging this truth, you open the door to unleashing the incredible potential of effective public communication. Underestimating your capacity to engage in presentations or address audiences might restrict both your professional advancements and personal achievements. Yaffe's (2018) research serves as a compelling reminder that the fear of public speaking can inhibit career progression to management by 15% and can even cut your earnings by 10%.

Quite simply, these essential skills are vital to your future, and the personal benefits can include:

- Improves your communication skills.
- Boosts your confidence and drives better personal satisfaction.
- Improves your critical thinking and problem-solving skills.
- Increases your ability to actively listen.
- Better management of conflict and developing negotiation skills.
- Influences decision-making and motivates change.
- Improves your social networking and career opportunities.

SOCIAL MEDIA
@RuthOshikanlu

'Public speaking allows us to convey information to many people, form connections, influence decisions, and motivate change; and is a vital skill for nurses at every level to have'.

| *I will* transform my fear into joy. | *I am* **excited** to practice the skill of public speaking. | *I feel* **comfortable** and **confident** when speaking and I **am** an **inspiring** speaker. |

Fig. 9.1   Quick affirmations.

So, let's get started on building that confidence right now! Start with the quick affirmations outlined in Fig. 9.1.

Practice saying these in the mirror every day, if possible. Alternatively, you can choose words that reflect how you would like to build your own confidence. This is also very effective when said aloud just before you need to speak publicly.

SOCIAL MEDIA
@GloStarsNHS

'Being able to advocate through public speaking is challenging. However, it is a fundamental skill set within Nursing. In our peer support work, we use it daily to advocate for staff well-being & to promote positive practice cultures. We've found team affirmations really help'!

Part of finding your voice is knowing and understanding what your style and public speaking philosophies are, and so, this is what we're going to explore next in this chapter.

What is your presenting style and philosophy?

In the world of social media and TED talks, you don't have to go far to find some incredible public speakers. Nelson Mandela, Martin Luther King Jr., Malala Yousafzai and Jane Goodall are all world-renowned for their public speaking abilities.

So, what makes these people great speakers? Some might suggest that certain people are born as natural public speakers; others would argue that exceptional speakers have been educated and trained in the art and skill of it. One thing we can probably all agree upon is that we can learn a great deal from astonishing and distinguished speakers.

In this chapter, I want to take the opportunity to draw attention to excellent public speakers who are nurses. The art of public speaking is carried through all walks of life, not simply with those on a media platform; remember that you are likely surrounded by exceptional presenters and speakers in your day-to-day communications. Perhaps you have not noticed them before, but now is your opportunity to start to actively listen and observe those around you who can help influence your style and presenting philosophy. This could be through larger events such as conferences, lectures or training, but it could also be during smaller day-to-day activities such as multidisciplinary team (MDT) meetings or handovers.

Think about those who communicate in a way that leaves you in awe. What is it about their delivery that you aspire to become?

_____

_____

_____

_____

SOCIAL MEDIA
@etaltraining

'Presenting with impact can be a key skill. Cast your mind back to a presentation you remember as brilliant and influenced you - ask yourself what is it that made it memorable? That presenter will have prepared well and practiced the skills'.

When it comes to inspiring nurse speakers, we are a profession filled with vast talent, from nurse author Christie Watson delivering keynote speeches in an authentic, compassionate and connecting way to Dame Elizabeth Anionwu, who eloquently fills a room with her knowledge, competence and thought-provoking questioning. There is so much we can learn from these great presenters and speakers to help facilitate our own growth in discovering our presenting style and philosophy.

Here is some top advice that I have sought to share with you from inspirational nurse speakers who have motivated my progression in public speaking:

'I think it is important to feel a little anxious when presenting - I still do. It means that the presentation really matters and that you want to do a good job and recognise the responsibility of presenting to others and getting it right. Also, a bit of adrenaline always helps you to think more clearly and talk more articulately - which is always a challenge for me!!

The other things that help me are:

- *To remember what I am passionate about (i.e., Being person/ people centered; leadership as enablement; bringing out the best in everyone, and the potential for people working together to shift mountains).*
- *Always try and link to the evidence base and different types of knowledge, whilst I always appreciate there are different ways of understanding knowledge and that all types of knowledge are important and complement each other.*
- *Be prepared when presenting new ideas and insights to persevere, as often at first, they are rejected/ criticized because they may be different to what people are used to. Eventually though the new ideas come into their own.*
- *I usually forewarn people before I say things that I know might be unpopular - this shows that I recognise the impact on others and that we might respectfully disagree about certain things, but I will always listen to the other argument and will think a lot about it.*

- I always try to evaluate and reflect on what I might do differently next time, inviting comments about how it could be better'.

Kim Manley, CBE, Emeritus Professor

- 'Understand who you are and your purpose, this will provide authenticity to your voice and will help you connect with the audience.
- Be honest in your message and mean it, being true to yourself and the spoken word lies at the centre of your moral compass and your True North. People will see and hear this.
- Show vulnerability, we all present various versions of ourselves, however, when you present the truest version of yourself on that stage/platform/floor this will resonate with those you are speaking to. It can be a very powerful for you and for them.
- Love what you do and love what you speak about. When you feel this inside you, it will transmit to others, and they will feel it too. How you make an audience feel will stay with them always.
- Believe in your story and message. If you don't believe in it, it becomes meaningless. It has to mean something to you if it does let that be seen and heard. The chances are it will resonate and mean something to others.
- If you are nervous, that's good. Use the energy, breathe in deeply and out and then remember this is not about you, this is about the purpose, who you are advocating for, who you are giving a voice to, who at this moment in time cannot have their voice heard'.

Professor Aisha Holloway, Professor of Nursing Studies, Co-Director and Programme Director of the Nursing Now Challenge

- *'One of the counter-intuitive ways of thinking about presenting with confidence is to remember it's not about you, it's about the audience you are there to serve - with the message(s) you want to share with them. When you frame it that way it enables you to get out of your own head and can help you convert your nervousness of getting it 'wrong' into a desire to share your enthusiasm and passion for your subject. Noted, nerves are normal and being in sinus tachycardia before you speak is too – just rebadge it as excitement!*

- *When speaking, remember you wouldn't listen to a piano for long if it only played one note, so vary the melody of your voice and that includes speeding up and slowing down your pace of delivery. Just as you don't want too many words on a PowerPoint, you don't have to fill every moment with sound either. So, if you have a key point you want to land, say it and then allow a few seconds of silence. This will give your audience time to process the points you've made and will add gravitas to your words.*

- *We connect through story and as Jonathan Gottschall wrote 'Even when the body goes to sleep, the mind stays up all night telling itself stories'. People will remember the stories you told and how you made them feel far more than the facts you shared.*

- *Engage in call and response; for instance, a question like, 'If you had 1,000 days to live, how many would you choose to spend in hospital?' is simple and easy to answer as it's invariably 'None'. It really engages the audience and makes them part of your presentation.*

- *Just as you want speakers to present well, the audience wishes you well too and you know you've served them when they think differently about what they thought before. What a good thing it is that it's about them not you!'*

Professor Brian Dolan, OBE, Director

'Great presenting within your work environment is all about you as the presenter being in a positive frame of mind. It is normal to be nervous when presenting so have a couple of techniques in your kitbag to settle your nerves beforehand. I sometimes take a couple of deep slow breaths and ground myself in the space where I am about to present. As part of your introduction, find something that connects you with the people you are speaking to – when you make a connection you can be your authentic self and be at your best. Do not worry that you do not know everything. You were asked to present for a reason and if you don't know something, that is okay – either someone in the audience will or you can go away and find out and feedback to the person later'.

Paul Vaughan, Deputy Director, Primary Care Nursing and NextGen Nurse

- 'Start and end with a meaningful and memorable story.
- Use slides to enhance understanding of your presentation by including catchy visuals and key points. Do not read the content verbatim.
- Engage your audience through gaming (charades, Jeopardy) and online polling platforms (example: poll everywhere)
- Leverage use of technology but have a back-up plan. Have a printout of your notes or handouts ready.
- And Practice. Practice. Practice!'

Rhoda Redulla, Director of Nursing Excellence & Magnet Recognition

'I try to tap into what people are really interested in by finding out what matters to them as a key priority to focus on so that the focus of a session is co-created with the people I am working with. Finding out what people are interested in and what makes them tick and enabling them to find out more about each other when

Continued

you are on a collaborative learning journey together is really important. It helps us to connect and find out more about each other to get the most out of the experience together.

As well as being robust, systematic and evidence based it is important to tap into people's creativity as not everyone learns at the same pace or in the same way so using visuals and creative methods can help overcome people's anxieties. So, I use poetry, imagery, self-tests and stories to help people to connect with what interests them and each other.

I don't like public speaking much and always feel anxious, so I like to use humour and a bit of drama to steady my nerves and to connect with others.

I build in process and impact evaluation into everything I do so that we are all looking together at what we are learning as we go sharing new insights and thinking about what difference this will make to our practice.

It is good to achieve a balance of ensuring you have a range of materials to meet people's needs so that each session is evidence based, creative and interesting with follow up reading. This creates a good holistic approach. So, I always have a session outline to work from to keep track of things that I may miss or are not needed but need to be revisited elsewhere. That also helps you to work out roles and timings when you are facilitating sessions with others and helps you to be clear about who is doing what when. It also means that if anything goes wrong the cofacilitator can pick up where you left off!'

Carrie Jackson, Associate Professor, Practice Transformation

'Prepare; there are very few folks who can spontaneously rise to their feet and deliver their own personal "I have a dream" speech. Work out what your absolute core message is and what you want people to remember, don't overdo facts or technical speak, know who your target audience is as your message will be crafted differently but don't overcomplicate or over think what you say. Be real and authentic - people quickly smell the BS and your passion (controlled so as not to be a rant which can be an immediate turn off) can be as powerful as the message you want to deliver. As uncomfortable and cringe inducing as it can be to listen back to yourself; do it - in private is fine! It will help you learn and refine. There will be cringes that are the result of cliches that you might want to avoid in future, but some cringes may be a barometer of your honesty and openness which can strengthen your message. Final point - never forget that you have been asked to speak because someone thinks you have something to say that needs to be heard and take confidence from that'.

Howard Catton, CEO, International Council of Nurses

- *'Keep your notes/presentation simple, do not over complicate key messages, or over engineer if you are using digital tools - less is more.*
- *Practice by yourself and/or with a trusted friend/colleague in advance – it's really good to hear out loud what you are saying.*
- *Be yourself and don't think it has to be perfect to win over your audience. Authenticity is key and none of us are infallible. If you make a mistake, take a deep breath, acknowledge it and then move on.*
- *Enjoy it - aim to both educate and entertain the audience and yourself – it's surprising how much the speaker can learn from the audience as well as the other way round.'*

Professor Lisa Bayliss-Pratt, Chief Academic Officer

Review the quotes. What are the top three things you are going to take forward to start feeling more confident in presenting information?

_____

_____

_____

_____

When you next hear or listen to a new public speaker, reflect on what you like and don't like about that person's delivery:

- What will you take forward into your practice?
- What will you not take forward into your own practice?
- Anything else worth noting?
- What actions do you need to take?

_____

_____

_____

_____

Presenting through pantomime

Human communication extends beyond spoken language, encompassing body language, gestures and facial expressions. 'Presenting through pantomime' is an expressive art form where individuals craft intricate narratives using their bodies' silent language. This technique transcends performance and becomes a metaphorical portal, allowing for creativity, subtlety and depth in communication. Pantomime resonates with our innate desire to share and connect, and it requires constant nurturing and improvement to thrive. As people's thinking and actions evolve, it is essential to nurture our communication skills to thrive. This section will delve into the mesmerising universe of pantomime, exploring its multifaceted dimensions and uncovering how it resonates with our innate human desire to share and connect. Treat your ability to speak and present like a houseplant—it must not only be maintained but nurtured to thrive. We must constantly work on our communication skills because the way people think and act is constantly changing.

SOCIAL MEDIA

@VickyCuthill

'It's really important...on so many levels - from presenting a case at an MDT, to passing on your knowledge in a teaching presentation to articulating a service development need to a senior manager...if we don't do this well, our collective voice is weaker'.

The distribution of voice and language, both verbal and nonverbal, has changed significantly over time and will continue to evolve (The Health Foundation, 2015). Communication needs to be relevant and appropriate to the time you are delivering it. For example, if I opened a presentation with 'Valorous aft'rnoon, welcometh to my presentation on shared decision making', I might get some odd looks passed back and forth (unless, of course, Shakespeare was the topic at hand). The point is, the way we speak matters, sometimes even more than the content at hand. If you struggle with the idea of standing up in front of a room of people and speaking, consider this: the Beyonce theory. Say what? That's right, the diva herself struggles with stage fright even after years of being an internationally renowned entertainer, and a way in which she has learnt to overcome this fear is by 'playing the presenter'. For Beyonce, she uses an alter ego called Sasha Fierce. Now I'm not saying you need to create a character for yourself, but think about who it is that is going to stand there and command the space, both online and in person.

When you have begun to understand who you are as a speaker, you can then get down to the really important stuff: your audience. Understanding the needs and desires of your audience is crucial to success. The best speakers in the world think about what their audience needs and less about what they personally need to be successful. In pantomimes, performers win over their audiences through their ability to engage and capture their interest. The performer must understand and read the reactions and behaviours of their audience in real time. This might vary between each performance because everyone is different; the same principle applies in presenting. This is why it's important to set ground rules and understand what it is your audience is seeking from your delivery at that moment; what is the goal? Are you teaching or motivating? What do they want to gain from being there? By being open, authentic and relentlessly you, you are moving past the need to please everyone and moving into a space of shared learning and participation; this can ultimately relieve the great pressure of presenting, and you might even start to enjoy public speaking.

TIPS TO IMPROVE YOUR PRESENTATION SKILLS

Learn to think on your feet

This activity will help you learn about your response mechanisms and help you to practice giving quick answers without overthinking to develop your ability to improvise and become more articulate on the spot.

- Use a random question generator online (found via all good search engines) to find a question.
- Time yourself for 1 minute and answer the question, recording it on your phone.
- Listen back and reflect on what you liked and didn't like about your impromptu answer.

Emphasis is everything

By overemphasising each word when we speak and focusing on driving consonants and vowels in sentences, we create fully audible diction, which helps us to deliver clearer and eloquent messaging to our listeners.

- You can improve your ability to do this by using classic tongue twisters or by repeating hard-to-say phrases such as 'red lorry, yellow lorry'.
- Say these phrases repeatedly and keep speeding up each time, making it harder until you are no longer able to say it clearly.
- Keep at this short exercise every day, and you will see a vast improvement in your diction and articulation.

Style of expression—speak with clarity and conciseness in your diction!

A great way to build clear and effective articulation of words is by practicing saying words in languages that you do not speak—seems odd, right? However, this method will help you to explore the pronunciation of words and sounds, and if you are feeling really bold, you could even practice this exercise through singing in languages you don't know.

Pausing is power!

This will help you to start to build stamina and to feel comfortable under pressure; in turn, this can help to reduce that nervous rush that we all inevitably feel when public speaking or presenting. This exercise also helps you to replace the typical 'umms' and 'ahhs' we use as gap fillers; a clear and confident presenter replaces them with strong pauses of clarity.

- Choose someone you trust, a family member, friend or colleague; start to talk about a topic you are passionate about or present some work that you have already written.
- Start this exercise off by delivering it as you would normally; then, the second time round, you are going to add in significant pauses. This WILL and should feel uncomfortable.
- Ask your observer to raise their hand when they want you to take a pause; encourage them to do this often and even in unusual places, not just between paragraphs but through sentences and even between single words.
- Work through the uncomfortable silence, and practice allowing yourself to gaze into the audience's eyes.

Build better self-awareness

You need to be aware of how you sound, e.g., volume, pace, pitch, body language, facial expressions as well as what word you use to enable you to identify the issues and the words used that may rob you of a confident and articulate delivery.

- Get your phone and video record yourself speaking about any topic of interest for 5 minutes—this should be unplanned and not scripted or overthought. Just go for it!

Continued

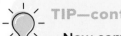

TIP—cont'd

- Now complete an auditory review; take your phone, turn the volume right up and press play, but don't watch the video footage. Just listen, and take notes on your vocal delivery.
  - How is my volume?
  - Am I rushing; am I pausing enough?
  - Is there emotion in my voice?
  - What are the sounds telling me?
  - Is my pitch and diction clear?
- Now complete a visual review; take your phone and turn off the volume completely so that there is no sound. Press play and just watch yourself.
  - Watch back your body language.
  - Notice your nonverbal behaviours.
  - Are you delivering the content through your movements? Does it correlate to your content messaging?
- Finally, transcribe your video: take a highlighter to your words and notice any nonwords or filler dialogue within your speaking.

Build dynamic range

Dynamic range in your delivery will make you a presenter who commands the attention of your audience. I have attended many keynote speeches in the past where I can't recall much detail of the contents but was somehow fully immersed and left feeling inspired and empowered simply by the charismatic delivery of the speaker. You, too, can develop this level of lasting impact by speaking with every single word FULLY announced. The more you practice this, the more natural it will start to become. We have all tried desperately to stay awake, with matchsticks in our eyes when someone is presenting in a monotone voice or is simply reading slides from the presentation to us. When people present like this and shy away from the delivery aspect of the presentation, it doesn't even matter if their content is distinction level; the delivery will leave no impact on the receiver. Giving life to your sentences as if it were a chat amongst friends gives authenticity and allows the audience to come on a journey with you through storytelling. This enables listeners to connect with you and your content.

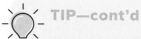

TIP—cont'd

- You can practice doing this at home simply by reading a book, magazine article or even a microwave meal packaging aloud. Do this in different pitches and ranges, have fun with it and give it character and a little pizzazz; you will be amazed at how this 'silliness' will lift your confidence to speak in a more dynamic way.

Increase your energy

An easy way to vamp up your energy while public speaking is to simply increase your volume.

- Start by scaling your normal speaking style out of 10. For example, I am generally a rather loud and somewhat irritating person, so I range casually (chatting with friends across the dinner table) at around a 6 out of 10.
- When speaking in a room full of people or presenting, you need to elevate your voice style and range at least two levels higher than in a casual setting. So, for me that would be delivering at a vocal level of 8 out of 10, this helps to project my voice and increases the energy of my delivery overall.

Feedback and reflection

A common mistake in developing presenting and public speaking skills is practicing in isolation. While there are many exercises you can work on alone, to really meet your full potential, you need to gain feedback from others. When practicing delivery alone, you are simply working methodically through your steps, essentially creating what you imagine to be the best version of delivery. However, what this doesn't do is account for the human factors of public speaking, the stage fright, the muttering to one another amongst the audience and the phone gazers.

By gaining feedback on our approach to delivery, we can start to understand the impression we give to others when speaking. This allows us greater insight into understanding our blind spots and creates a basis for personal action improvements to be made. The seminal Johari Window Model of Interpersonal Awareness by Luft and Ingham (1955) is a great tool to review and understand our relationships with ourselves

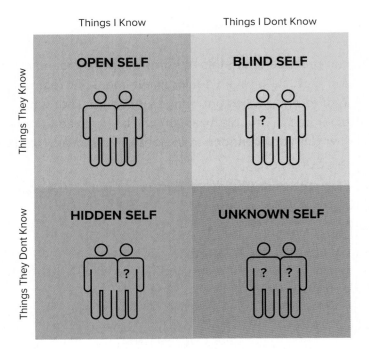

Fig. 9.2   Johari's window.

and others. We encourage you to search online and read what it is all about, and next time you present, complete the Johari Window model (Fig. 9.2) to better identify areas for improvement. By opening ourselves up to recognise our blind spots, we can build upon our self-awareness and emotional intelligence and create purposeful self-improvement goals.

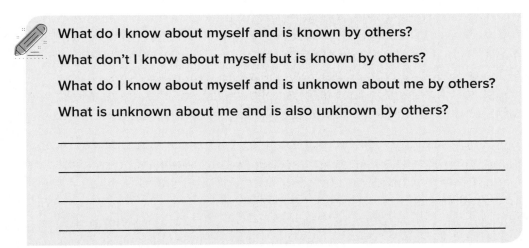

What do I know about myself and is known by others?

What don't I know about myself but is known by others?

What do I know about myself and is unknown about me by others?

What is unknown about me and is also unknown by others?

Lived experiences of nursing students—you are not alone

When it comes to public speaking of any form, most people experience an instant spiral of panic. It's important that we learn and grow from our experiences, both good and bad, and not allow imposter syndrome to take over residency in our future thoughts and actions (see Chapters 1 and 11). To better understand and know how we can start to take back control of our emotions and self-doubts, we must first practice self-compassion. You may be familiar with our frenemy perfectionism; well, when it comes to delivering work through public speaking such as assessment-based presentations, we need to disrupt the cycle of negative rumination and those thoughts we have around, such as 'I'm just not good at…'. Presenting is a complex skill set that everyone can develop, and anything worthwhile takes time and investment to gain confidence and competence. Have you ever found yourself holding back from applying for a new job or taking advantage of an exciting opportunity because of the fear of failure or feeling overwhelmed by the application process? Maybe you've had thoughts like, 'I don't have the necessary skills' or 'I'm not knowledgeable enough'. However, it's important to remember that you've already come this far because of your willingness to be open and vulnerable and your acceptance of the idea of learning and growth. A growth mindset is beneficial in different areas of life, allowing us to excel in our academic pursuits, careers and personal relationships (Yeager and Dweck, 2012; Dweck and Blackwell, 2016).

Self-awareness can be enhanced through reflection. By examining our experiences and situations in a reflective manner, we can gain a realistic understanding of our performance and identify areas for improvement. Over the years, I have spoken to numerous nursing students from diverse backgrounds who have faced similar challenges when it comes to public speaking. The following are real case studies of nursing students who have shared their experiences.

CASE STUDY

I have been involved in group work with other students where we were aware of having different approaches but had done our best to work together and agree on a plan. The role of spokesperson

Continued

was 'sprung' on me at the last minute, and our group was the last to give feedback, which meant that a lot of the other groups had already put forward most of the ideas we had come up with. We had also discussed a lot of ideas, but not written them all down, so looking at our document on the screen, we hadn't appeared to have done much!

I felt like a rabbit in headlights and struggled to put my sentences together properly. In my head, I was feeling judged by both the lecturer and the more confident students who had already fed back. The more my inner voice was criticising me, the more tongue-tied I became. The rest of my group was very supportive, as they were aware of how much I hate speaking to large groups, particularly without a script or plan.

Next time we have group work, I will make sure we agree upfront who is the spokesperson, and then if it's me, I can take separate notes that make sense to me. I'm also aware that presenting to a large group is a skill that I will need to develop.

Emerson Mironescu, a first-year children's nursing student

Emerson's reflection highlights the challenges and dynamics that can arise within group work settings. The experience underscores the importance of proactive planning and communication within groups, including designating roles in advance to distribute responsibilities effectively. It also highlights the realisation that public speaking is a skill requiring development and practice.

SOCIAL MEDIA
@Kimxx060928

'We encourage speaking in groups and presenting in our undergraduate programme. Public speaking doesn't come naturally to some, and I think as a profession we have to support students to build confidence not just to speak publicly but to engage with audiences (whomever they are)'.

CASE STUDY

'Hello, my name is Honor' is a sentence I have said many times without a second thought. Put me in front of some lecturers with a marking grid, tell me it's a presentation and I forget my name. As trainee nursing associates, we were told that much like nursing, presenting was going to be part of our degree. Yet when I embarked on my journey back into education, I couldn't even hold my hand up in lectures and say the answers without my voice shaking and the blood draining from my face. Fast forward to my bachelor of science in nursing, and I received my highest grade ever for a presentation. How did I get there? I really had no idea until I sat down to write this reflection. So welcome to my short story of how I overcame the fear of presenting from the perspective of a nursing associate lacking in confidence.

My first presentation was not exactly one to shout home about. I had my lowest mark to date, I couldn't read my presentation notes, I hated the subject and I am pretty sure a tear or two slipped out halfway through. When seeking advice from my lecturer, she asked me, 'Did you prepare?' What did she mean? I looked up from my notes I had taken as if to say... 'I have clearly prepared because I have notes in my hand!' Then I looked down at my notes, and I had no idea whatsoever what I meant by them. Yes, I had researched the topic and had provided arguments for evidence-based practice, but when I stood in front of my audience with just these things, I simply froze.

The next time I was asked to present was in front of aspirant nursing associates. Personally, I think one of the great things about healthcare roles is that, really, we are presenting all the time, whether it be health education in front of patients and relatives, ongoing education for colleagues or even pitching quality improvement to the chief executive of the hospital. So, when asked to present in front of colleagues, I thought, 'I know enough about this topic; I don't need notes.' Boy, was I wrong. I left that Zoom meeting feeling deflated and as if I had so much more to offer in terms of advice and guidance for the people wanting to go down the same path as me. Funnily enough, after this opportunity, I had another chance to speak on behalf of the trust. Once again, I didn't feel I could offer as much as I wanted to when presenting due to anxiety and leaving little to no time for preparation.

Continued

CASE STUDY—cont'd

See a theme here? I didn't until I embarked on the next stage of my nursing degree. Enter one of my proudest moments in my many years of education. Next up was a level 6 group presentation, something I suddenly felt more people were reliant on me to do well in. Not only did I have more experience presenting on my side but I had also gained some confidence. That did not mean that I felt able to stand in front of an audience who quite clearly knew more about the topic than me. Fuelled by my group and my previous experiences, I sought out an alternative way to present. On the day of this presentation, I felt that I had locked down my arguments and research methods, but to show my markers that I understood what I was talking about, I needed to prove that I had understood just that. I read my notes hundreds of times to ensure that I knew what they meant. I needed to rehearse so that I knew what was coming up next and so that it flowed smoothly. I practiced in front of a mirror, my phone, my friends and my dog. Anyone who would listen and anyone who wouldn't. I became confident in what I was talking about, and I became an expert in the very small portion of the presentation that was mine. I despised the topic, but I made it mine, and it became my passion for those weeks of rehearsing. I had cue cards that I had learnt front and back, meaning that I was prompting myself instead of just reading from a piece of paper. In turn, this meant that I was able to engage with the audience, albeit a small audience.

I guess what I am trying to say is that preparation is key and that as cliché as it sounds, you really cannot practice enough.

Honor Govan, RNA, third-year adult nursing student

Honor's story reinforces the timeless adage that 'preparation is key'. The journey from trembling nerves to confident expertise serves as a testament to the power of practice, resilience and the willingness to learn and adapt. Honor's path exemplifies the transformation from a tentative presenter to a knowledgeable and confident communicator, embodying the spirit of growth and self-improvement.

SOCIAL MEDIA

@LorenaHall77

'Most important is know your subject. Confidence will be high then... Nerves are natural'.

@LisaHyattRN

'I think it's important to remember that even those who stand in front of classes regularly are still nervous. It's all about practice. I find Amy Cuddy's TED Talks about power posing really helpful; your posture can actually give you a boost of courage'.

CASE STUDY

I recently had to participate in a group presentation for a university assessment. The topic was shared decision-making, and we had to collaborate as a group to prepare and present our information to a panel. We had a maximum of 40 minutes for our presentation, with the panel asking follow-up questions on each other's slides. The result would be a shared grade. I have limited experience of public speaking, and it is something that does not come naturally to me. I found the process quite daunting. I often feel nervous before public speaking and an assessment, and this exercise combined the two! I wanted to ensure that I did the best I could so I would not let the other group members down. Luckily, the others had a similar work ethic, so we were successful in preparing our work together.

When it came to the presentation itself, I felt the usual exam stress feelings—racing heart, butterflies in my tummy, feeling flushed and having clammy hands. I had to force myself not to read word for word from my cue cards, remember to refer to my prepared PowerPoint slides and make eye contact with the panel. Having the other group members next to me made me feel more comfortable than if I had been presenting individually.

I found that working in a group provided opportunities for collaborative and shared learning, with everyone bringing different

Continued

CASE STUDY—cont'd

ideas and clinical experiences together. This resulted in a more diverse presentation that I would not have been able to produce individually. This was particularly useful during the follow-up questions when we could build upon and contribute to developing someone else's answer. I was fortunate that my group members all worked together in a respectful way, sharing the work evenly. This could have been an area of stress if it had not been the case.

From my very first placement, I have had to present patients in MDT meetings. I find these nerve-wracking, but if I have the information in front of me and have been able to prepare, they feel more manageable. As I have developed as a student, I believe my presenting skills have improved, but this is because I have more confidence in the content area rather than from practicing presenting skills. I have found that the more I know about a topic, I can speak more naturally and confidently and can present with more ease overall.

Alex Valentine, second-year mental health nursing student

Alex's experience demonstrates the significance of having confidence in the subject you are delivering, which not only facilitates a smoother and more confident delivery but also elevates the overall quality of the presentation. The collaborative essence of the task vividly demonstrates the potency of combined expertise and the benefits derived from distributing workloads collectively. While refining presentation skills remains crucial, the foundational knowledge and self-assuredness within the subject matter assume a pivotal role in presenting persuasively and with confidence.

NMC

THE NMC SAYS

8.2 'Maintain effective communication with colleagues'.
8.6 'Share information to identify and reduce risk'.

SOCIAL MEDIA

@ Helen_Friz

'Even if not presenting something, being able to speak clearly, professionally & with good enunciation is important at meetings, interviews etc if you want to be treated credibly'

CASE STUDY

I had to present in a group as part of my Approaches to Research Methods, Appraisal and Application module. We had to deliver a PowerPoint presentation on a subject called 'What impact has nursing staff shortages had on the quality of student nurse's placement experience'. When creating the group presentation, each team member came together to complete their own part, and the entire presentation came together much quicker.

The feedback received indicated that there was some uncertainty about the research process, so I could have done further reading on this, and some aspects of the presentation could have also been explained more clearly, for example, participant selection and data collection to demonstrate understanding of the research process followed.

Public speaking and presentation are a necessary and important part of nursing. It allows nurses to impart knowledge to educate and persuade colleagues to adopt new ways of working and engage service users and colleagues in clinical projects.

Joanna Rosa Mendes, third-year adult nursing student

Joanna's experience emphasises the essential role that public speaking and presentation skills play in the nursing field. By honing these skills, nurses are equipped to disseminate evidence-based knowledge effectively, influence colleagues to embrace innovative approaches and actively engage both service users and coworkers in clinical initiatives.

'My advice for presenting with confidence:

- *Make eye contact*
- *Keep an open posture*
- *Use gestures*
- *Eliminate filler words*
- *Take time to pause*
- *Vary your pace'*

Joanna Rosa Mendes, third-year adult nursing student

THE NMC SAYS

9. 'Share your skills, knowledge and experience for the benefit of people receiving care and your colleagues'.

SOCIAL MEDIA
@ KWebbNurse

'#WeStudentNurse Presenting case studies, advocacy for patients, teaching formally & informally, all are enhanced by proper training. I use my PGCE skills frequently. Never forget as a professional that improving communication skills improves care & patient outcomes!'

Enhancing nursing care

As a nursing student, it is not just academic presentations but also, and more importantly, clinical experiences in placement which require effective presentation of information. This ensures compassionate and safe person-centred care. In some situations, clear and efficient communication is absolutely essential. You will come across various communication tools during your nursing education, but, arguably, the SBAR tool will be the most valuable. It is a structured communication technique widely used in healthcare settings and designed to improve the transfer of critical information between healthcare professionals (Advancing Quality Alliance (Aqua), 2021). Research indicates that patient safety is increased with SBAR use, especially when used as a structure for telephone communication (Müller et al., 2018). SBAR stands for situation, background, assessment and recommendation. As you can see in Fig. 9.3, using the SBAR tool helps you stay organised and focused and ensures that crucial information is not overlooked. This is what promotes patient safety, enhancing the overall quality of care and significantly improving collaboration among healthcare professionals (Park, 2020). Key points of care where the SBAR tool can be used include:

- Handovers during shift changes or when transferring patient care to another nurse to communicate essential patient information accurately and concisely.
- Consultations and referrals to present the patient concern and seek appropriate information and assistance recommendations.
- Interprofessional communication, when working with other healthcare professionals, helps foster effective communication and reduces the risk of misunderstandings.
- Reporting or escalation of concerns to other or more other senior healthcare staff.
- In emergency or time-sensitive situations to ensure that vital information is communicated quickly and efficiently to the appropriate team members.

The SBAR tool boosts confidence in presenting information by promoting clarity, standardisation and professionalism. It will empower you as a nursing student and as an experienced nurse to communicate more effectively, ultimately leading to improved patient outcomes.

Situation

First, introduce yourself and where you're from and provide a concise overview of the current situation. Include the reason for communication, and patient's relevant identifiers. Be specific about the current concern that requires attention

Example: 'This is Nursing Student Smith calling to report a change in Mrs Johnson's condition. She is a 65-year-old female with a history of hypertension. She has a sudden onset of shortness of breath and chest pain.'

Background

Here, present essential contextual information about the patient's health, wellbeing or welfare, diagnoses and recent events that may be contributing to the current issue. Provide a brief overview of current medications, recent tests or interventions, referrals.

Example: 'Mrs Johnson was admitted 3 days ago for uncontrolled hypertension. She is on a beta-blocker and an ACE inhibitor. Her recent echocardiogram showed a decreased ejection fraction.'

Assessment

Next you describe your objective observations and assessments of the patient's issue. In a clinical setting this may include vital signs, physical exam findings and any relevant lab or test results.

Example: 'Currently, Mrs Johnson's heart rate is 110 beats per minute, blood pressure is 160/90 mmHg, respiratory rate is 24 breaths per minute, and oxygen saturation is 88% on room air. She appears anxious and is using accessory muscles to breathe.'

Recommendation

This is where you offer your suggestions or requests for the next steps in the patient's care. Be clear and specific about what you think needs to happen to address the situation.

Example: 'Considering Mrs Johnson's symptoms and decreased oxygen saturation, I recommend administering supplemental oxygen, obtaining an ECG, notifying the duty doctor, including preparing for a possible transfer to ITU.'

Fig. 9.3   SBAR components and example.

Maybe you have learnt about or used the SBAR tool in simulation at university or observed it being used in placement or, indeed, a situation where you think it should have been used. What are your reflections on its use? What are the key things you need to remember when you use it next or for the first time?

_____

_____

_____

_____

Reflect on any non-patient-related situations when you had to speak in public. Maybe it was group work, a presentation in class or promoting yourself in an interview or your peers' views in university committee. How can you apply your learning above to these types of scenarios?

_____

_____

_____

_____

CONCLUSION

Presenting with confidence is a concept that many nurses struggle with; nearly all of us will experience some imposter syndrome throughout our studies and careers. This chapter has focused on building confidence in public speaking, as this will not only improve your ability to present but will also allow you to develop a range of communication skills that you can apply to your day-to-day work. We have explored the importance of gaining confidence and finding our voice in the classroom and beyond. We have identified how communication is fundamental to living the values of the NMC (2018) code, and the chapter has set out ways in which you can continue to practice building your skillset to present with confidence. Remember it's okay to be nervous; just use that energy to reframe your perspective to that of excitement to learn and grow.

Now you have finished this chapter. Please make notes on what you have learned.

_____

_____

_____

_____

_____

_____

_____

_____

_____

_____

_____

_____

_____

_____

_____

_____

_____

_____

_____

_____

_____

_____

_____

REFERENCES

Black, R. (2019) *Glossophobia (fear of public speaking): Are you glossophobic?* Available at https://www.psycom.net/glossophobia-fear-of-public-speaking (Accessed 27 July 2023).

Dweck, C. and Blackwell, L. (2016) 'Growth mindset feedback tool'. Mindset Works. Available at: http://www.mindsetworks.com/FileCenter/MM3J5lO126930FPPC4TD.pdf (Accessed 3 June 2023).

Furmark, T., Tillfors, M., Everz, P.O., Marteinsdottir, I., Gefvert, O. and Fredrikson, M. (1999) 'Social phobia in the general population: prevalence and sociodemographic profile'. *Social Psychiatry and Psychiatric Epidemiology*, 34(8), pp. 416–424. (Accessed 03 December 2022).

Grieve, R., Woodley, J., Hunt, S.E. and McKay, A. (2021) 'Student fears of oral presentations and public speaking in higher education: a qualitative survey', *Journal of Further and Higher Education*, 45(9), pp. 1281–1293. doi:10.1080/0309877x.2021.1948509.

Luft, J., & Ingham, H. (1955) The Johari window, a graphic model of interpersonal awareness. Proceedings of the Western Training Laboratory in Group Development, 246, 2014–03.

Müller, M., Jürgens, J., Redaèlli, M., Klingberg, K., Hautz, W.E. and Stock, S. (2018) 'Impact of the communication and patient hand-off tool SBAR on patient safety: A systematic review', *BMJ Open*, 8(8), p. e022202. Available at: https://doi.org/10.1136/bmjopen-2018-022202.

Advancing Quality Alliance (Aqua) (2021) *SBAR communication tool – situation, background, assessment, recommendation*. Available at: https://aqua.nhs.uk/wp-content/uploads/2023/07/qsir-sbar-communication-tool.pdf (Accessed 22 October 2023).

Nursing and Midwifery Council (NMC) (2018) The code: Professional standards of practice and behaviour for nurses, midwives and nursing associates [online]. *London: Nursing and Midwifery Council*. Available at: https://www.nmc.org.uk/standards/code/ (Accessed 10 November 2022).

Park, L.J. (2020) 'Using the SBAR handover tool', *British Journal of Nursing,* 29(14), pp. 812–813. Available at: https://doi.org/10.12968/bjon.2020.29.14.812.

The Health Foundation (2015) *Using communications approaches to spread improvement. A practical guide to help you effectively communicate and spread your improvement work* [online]. Available at: https://www.health.org.uk/sites/default/files/UsingCommunicationsApproaches_revised%2 0page.pdf (Accessed 27 November 2022).

Yaffe, P. (2018) 'Banishing the fear of public speaking', *Ubiquity*, 2018, pp. 1–15. doi:10.1145/3281453

Yeager, D.S. and Dweck, C.S. (2012) 'Mindsets that promote resilience: when students believe that personal characteristics can be developed', *Educational Psychologist*, 47(4), pp. 302–314. Available at: https://doi.org/10.1080/00461520.2012.722805.

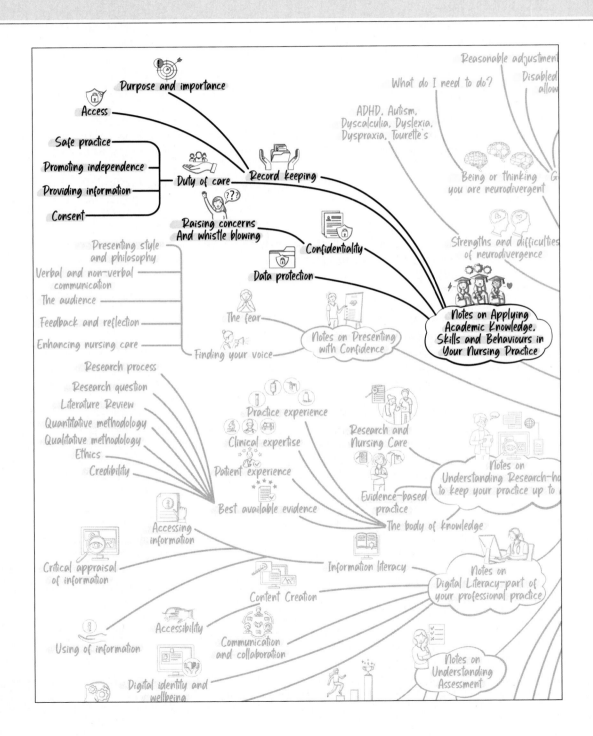

Purpose and importance

Access

Safe practice
Promoting independence
Providing information
Consent

Duty of care

Record keeping

Raising concerns
And whistle blowing

Confidentiality

Data protection

Reasonable adjustment

What do I need to do?

Disabled
allow

ADHD, Autism,
Dyscalculia, Dyslexia,
Dyspraxia, Tourette's

Being or thinking
you are neurodivergent

Strengths and difficulties
of neurodivergence

Notes on Applying
Academic Knowledge,
Skills and Behaviours in
Your Nursing Practice

Presenting style
and philosophy
Verbal and non-verbal
communication
The audience
Feedback and reflection
Enhancing nursing care

The fear

Finding your voice

Notes on Presenting
with Confidence

Research process
Research question
Literature Review
Quantitative methodology
Qualitative methodology
Ethics
Credibility

Practice experience

Clinical expertise

Patient experience

Best available evidence

Accessing
information

Research and
Nursing Care

Evidence-based
practice

The body of knowledge

Notes on
Understanding Research—ho
to keep your practice up to

Critical appraisal
of information

Information literacy

Content Creation

Notes on
Digital Literacy—part of
your professional practice

Using of information

Accessibility

Communication
and collaboration

Notes on
Understanding
Assessment

Digital identity and
wellbeing

NOTES ON APPLYING ACADEMIC KNOWLEDGE, SKILLS AND BEHAVIOURS IN YOUR NURSING PRACTICE

Catherine Forward (she/her)

INTRODUCTION

Ensuring you prepare for practice and undertake your placements in a safe and professional way is an important part of your nursing programme. Whilst learning new skills and caring for different patients as part of a multidisciplinary team, you will be required to demonstrate your understanding of the nursing role and responsibilities as a student and future registrant. As outlined in Chapter 6, your competencies, professional values and behaviours will be assessed against the future nurse standards as set out by the Nursing and Midwifery Council (NMC) (2018a). These standards are in place to protect the public and ensure that nurses are accountable for their practice and can deliver safe, effective and compassionate care. Maintaining and demonstrating these standards will be required as part of your revalidation with the NMC once you are qualified (NMC, 2023a).

This chapter will focus on record-keeping as a key part of nursing care and how to make sure that your documentation is good quality, accurate and efficient in your own practice. It will also consider the consequences of poor record-keeping. It will examine duty of care and how it contributes to safe practice and promotes independence for your patients. Consent and confidentiality will also be discussed in this chapter to ensure an understanding of the legal duties and responsibilities of the registered nurse. Finally, your responsibilities, in relation to data protection and what to do when you have concerns, will be considered to ensure that you are delivering safe and effective care.

SOCIAL MEDIA
@TeresaLean1

'We need to ensure that we support all staff to attain the right experience and qualifications to maintain patient safety'.

RECORD–KEEPING

NMC

THE NMC SAYS

1.8 'Write accurate, clear, legible records and documentation'.

What is the purpose of record-keeping, and why is it important?

At some point in your training, you will hear the phrase 'If it's not written down, it didn't happen'. This might be shared by a tutor in the classroom or your placement supervisor or assessor. It is good advice worth noting, as it protects you as well as your patients. It is a clear reminder that good record-keeping is an essential part of being a nurse, as well as a legal requirement (Andrews and St. Aubyn, 2015). As the NMC (2018a) explains, records must be accurate, clear and legible. Written records provide evidence that care has been delivered; they demonstrate and help create continuity of patient care and should make sense to others reading them in your absence. As a member of the wider healthcare team, nursing students will be asked to contribute to record-keeping under supervision, so it is important to give time to this task and ensure you are contributing to effective care. It is also important to note that a registered nurse should not be countersigning notes unless they have witnessed the care or can validate that the activity has taken place (NHS Professionals, 2018).

Records include (but are not limited to):

- Handwritten and electronic patient records
- Handover sheets and admission, discharge and transfer checklists
- Medication charts and vital signs observations
- Text messages used in the course of professional work
- Reports, including test and laboratory results
- Patients' assessment sheets such as nutrition or pressure area care assessment.

(NHS Professionals, 2018)

Good-quality record-keeping involves clear written communication that explains what care has been delivered, and it must be completed as soon as possible after the event. This increases the reliability of the record and minimises errors as well as enhancing credibility and reliability of the record as evidence (Griffith, 2016). Appropriate sharing of information is important within a healthcare team to ensure continuity of care. There are many demands on the time of a nurse, and unfortunately, record-keeping is sometimes viewed as a chore that is not given enough attention at the end of a shift. This approach may lead to increased risk of harm to our patients, and it is important that the time for quality record-keeping is protected.

'Documentation is the foundation and the key to good nursing practice. It underpins everything you do and makes certain you have the evidence of the care you have given. Patients trust us to ensure that we look after them, providing the right care and they are putting their care in our hands. We must always respect that and put ourselves in their shoes. Documenting carefully and completely ensures that the person who cares for that patient after we do is able to maintain the patient's journey'.

Abigail Payne, ward sister.

If record-keeping is poor, it will have a negative impact on patient care and decision-making because good records allow us to identify problems and address them (Stevens and Pickering, 2010). Furthermore, it could result in registrants receiving sanctions from the NMC or being removed from the register altogether, examples of which are outlined in Fig. 10.1. Sanctions are imposed to protect the public and maintain confidence, as well as ensure that standards are upheld by the profession. Therefore, it is of paramount importance that record-keeping is given the attention required as part of effective and safe practice delivery. Record writing should be approached as if the record will be

Examples of poor record-keeping practice	NMC sanctions and outcomes
Falsification of records	In **2020**, a health visitor was struck off the register for recording that they had completed a looked-after child review when they had not done so and for recording a child's weight when they had not taken it. It was also noted that their electronic records were inconsistent with their paper diary and that they had cut and pasted from previous records when undertaking assessments (**NMC, 2020**).
Accessing records inappropriately	An **NHS** worker was sacked and another reprimanded for inappropriately accessing the records of singer Ed Sheeran (Embury-Dennis, **2018**).
Failure to record documents in patient notes and to escalate concerns	In **2023**, a registered nurse was given a conditions of practice order following allegations of failure to record documents and to escalate concerns raised. In its report, the **NMC** stated that this approach illustrates 'the importance of maintaining public confidence in the profession and will send to the public and the profession a clear message about the standards of practice required of a registered nurse'. (**NMC, 2023b**)
Accessing records without legal or clinical reason	A nurse was removed from the register by the **NMC**, prosecuted by the information commissioner, fined and dismissed from their job after they were found to have accessed over **3000** records without legal or clinical reason in a 2-year period (**Smith, 2016**). Their employer described it as a *serious breach of trust*.
Accessing records of family or friends	A registered nurse was referred to the **NMC** by her employer in **2023** for inappropriately accessing **48** patient records, including her own and that of her baby (**NMC, 2023c**). The **NMC** concluded that her fitness to practice was impaired and stated that 'nurses occupy a position of privilege and trust in society and are expected at all times to be professional and to respect the confidentiality of patients'.

Fig. 10.1   Examples of sanctions and outcomes imposed by the NMC following poor record keeping practice.

relied upon in court to demonstrate that you have discharged your duty of care (Griffith, 2016).

When accessing patient records, it is important to only do so if you are involved in the care of that patient. There have been occasions where electronic records have been inappropriately accessed and read by people who are not involved in the patient's care (Griffith, 2018). It is important that it is understood that this is unprofessional behaviour that will have serious consequences.

When to access records and when not to

An important consideration when accessing patient records is why you are accessing them and whether or not you should be. You should not access the records of patients whose care you are not involved in. It is not acceptable to look up the records of friends or relatives. As Fig. 10.1 shows, you owe a duty of confidentiality to all those who are receiving care. Accessing records without cause is a breach of people's right to privacy and confidentiality, which could result in sanctions from the NMC for breaching the NMC code (2018) or the loss of your registration and your job.

NMC

THE NMC SAYS

'As a nurse, midwife, or nursing associate, you owe a duty of confidentiality to all those who are receiving care. This includes making sure that they are informed about their care and that information about them is shared appropriately. To achieve this, you must:

5.1. respect a person's right to privacy in all aspects of their care.
5.2. make sure that people are informed about how and why information is used and shared by those who will be providing care'.

TIP

- Use a systematic approach to ensure all information is included, and include details regarding how consent was obtained.
- Complete record-keeping contemporaneously (at the time or very soon afterward).
- Identify risks and problems and the steps taken to deal with them.
- Be accurate and factual without falsification.
- Do not use unnecessary abbreviations or jargon.
- If handwriting notes, use black ink and sign and date them.
- Any handwritten errors should be neatly crossed out with a single line so it is still legible; no Tipp-Ex.
- Ensure notes are kept securely, and if using electronic records, do not share your password.
- Only access notes for patients whose care you are directly involved with.

DUTY OF CARE

When discussing what good record-keeping includes, it has been explained that it is important to show that you have discharged your duty of care. This means that you have delivered care which meets the standards required, and it is a legal obligation that applies to you and those that you work within healthcare. The NMC's responsibility is to keep the public safe, and therefore, nurses, midwives and nursing associates should always follow the NMC code (2018) and other NMC guidance, including their publication 'Enabling Professionalism' (NMC 2023d).

What is a duty of care?

When being cared for by a nurse or health professional, patients should be able to trust the people involved with their health and well-being. They should be treated equally, with dignity and respect, and a good standard of care should be provided. There is also the requirement to avoid acts or omissions (failure to act) that can be predicted that would cause injury or harm (Peate, 2017). This is the professional duty of care. It is a responsibility you have to the people whose care you are delivering or involved with. It is different from the relationship you have with family and friends and is not an obligation you can opt out of. Part of your responsibility includes speaking out if you are unable to offer the best possible standard of care or if you have any concerns. Raising concerns will ensure that you and the healthcare team provide the best possible standard of care.

There are many ways in which you can maintain your standards of practice. These include keeping your knowledge and skills up to date and maintaining accurate and comprehensive records.

Can you think of other ways in which you can maintain your standards of practice as a nursing student and when you have qualified?

_____

_____

_____

_____

When you are a nursing student, your placement area must fulfil certain criteria to ensure that they deliver their duty of care as a learning environment and can provide 'safe and effective learning experiences'. The NMC clearly outlines the required standards that your placement area must achieve (NMC, 2019). These are outlined in Fig. 10.2.

What can I expect from my placement experiences?

- An overview of what to expect from your learning and assessment
- Relevant inductions and information
- A safe and effective learning experience
- Support from the right people
- Supernumerary and protected learning time
- Evidence-based, objective and fair assessments
- Reasonable adjustments (if applicable)
- **(NMC, 2019)**

Fig. 10.2 **What to expect from your placement experience.**

If you are a nursing apprentice, your employer also has a duty of care towards you as an employee. This will also be the case for registrants once employed. It is their responsibility to provide the appropriate training and equipment for your role and clearly outline your responsibilities in that role. It is important that you only undertake tasks that are within your scope of practice and competence, both as a nursing student and registrant. If you cannot undertake a task, you must highlight this and explain why.

How does a duty of care contribute to safe practice?

A duty of care (see Figure 10.3) applies to all types of healthcare settings but is particularly important in settings where at-risk patients with support needs, who are most in danger of harm or abuse, are cared for.

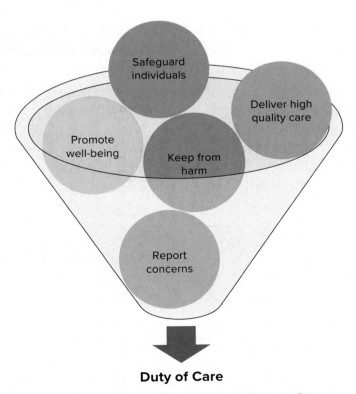

Duty of Care

Fig. 10.3   **Duty of care: things to consider.**

Completing individual person-centred care plans and undertaking risk assessments are examples of ways in which you are contributing to safe practice and fulfilling your duty of care. Challenging the practice of others, when necessary, is also an indirect way of empowering individuals.

CASE STUDY

When Gemma, a second-year adult nursing student, undertook her first placement, she was placed on a medical ward. She noticed a patient who had not been eating much food when they were given their meal tray and knew from handover that they had Parkinson's disease. Gemma decided to sit and chat with them and asked them how they were getting on. She thought about offering to feed them but felt nervous about doing that, as it seemed that they wanted to do it themselves but were struggling with holding their cutlery. Gemma decided to talk to her supervisor and asked if there was anything they could do to help. Her supervisor showed Gemma how to let the occupational therapist (OT) who visits the ward know, and the OT then arranged for the patient to have some adapted cutlery and crockery.

The supervisor highlighted to Gemma that this was an example of carrying out her 'duty of care' because she had considered their well-being, and it is important to ensure your patients are able to eat and drink. Gemma had just thought it was just 'the right thing to do', but talking about it with her supervisor gave her a better understanding of what a duty of care involves. Getting suitable cutlery and crockery arranged for the patient promoted their independence, and eating well helped their recovery and was good-quality care. Gemma had realised that if the patient couldn't eat properly, then they would have become more unwell, and it would have taken longer for them to be discharged home.

Promoting independence

When planning and delivering care, it is important that the client or individual's independence is promoted. People should be supported and encouraged to care for themselves, make their own decisions and be valued and recognised as an individual. Feeling in control of their lives and well-being can be transformative, and having choice will help to optimise an individual's physical and mental health (NHS England, 2017). Patients may make decisions that you do not personally agree with, but you must respect their opinions and promote individual choice.

'Following my strokes, when I was 26, I was unable to dress myself, wash myself, clean my teeth, brush my hair, shave my legs, do any of the personal care things I used to be able to do, especially in the first few weeks. I had to have that all done for me by nurses. Slowly, as I started to build some mobility, they helped me to do these things for myself. It would have been quicker for them to continue doing it for me but instead, they started to prompt me and remind me how to do things for myself. They would be there for safety but were constantly promoting my independence by showing me ways to work around my new mobility issues and lack of use of my hand. They were really good at teaching me how I could get clothes on with one sided weakness and to wash my hair and clean my teeth using one hand. Over a short amount of time, their help meant I could do these things for myself with this new disability. I really appreciated that. I was in hospital for a long time after my strokes and surgery, but it meant I could be alone doing those things again and it gave me the fighting spirit to try new things independently and work out ways around things, using one hand'.

Jo Vincent, *expert by experience*

Providing information

Another important aspect which promotes independence as part of our duty of care is to ensure our patients receive all the information they need to make informed decisions and can consent to treatment.

Different patients also have different developmental, linguistic and cultural needs, and these should be respected and promoted. For example, accessing written information about their care, in their own language, ensures accessibility whilst also promoting equality and addressing health inequalities.

CONSENT

'Consent is imperative. I have learnt over the years that gaining consent is also gaining the patient's trust for what you do, to what you write, and who you speak to, even other healthcare professionals. Never make assumptions and always document consent clearly. Remember, consent can be withdrawn at any time so always revisit this with your patient'.

Amanda Corr, prison nurse

What is informed consent?

When working as a nursing student and future nurse, understanding the importance of consent and the rationale behind the principles is imperative. To consent is to allow something or give permission for an action to happen. In relation to healthcare, it is a patient's right to decide about and agree to their care or treatment once they have the information to enable that decision and the time to consider the information (Avery, 2013). There is no requirement for consent to be provided in a set way: all are valid. However, written consent provides evidence and is preferred for certain procedures. Having said that, it is important to be aware that being in a written format does not automatically make the consent valid if the patient has not received adequate information to make an informed decision. In law, any adult who is mentally competent to consent has the right of action in the civil courts to sue for trespass (battery) to the person if consent was not obtained. Where consent was acquired but there was inadequate information provided, then there may be a case for negligence if there was a breach of a duty of care to inform the patient (Dimond, 2011).

What makes consent valid?

As well as requiring all the information relevant to make the decision informed, consent must also be freely given without duress. The adult providing consent must also have the capacity to make decisions, and being able to consent means that there is also a right to refuse treatment. In healthcare and law, it is presumed that adults are competent and have the capacity to make decisions. Any doubts or concerns about a patient's capacity should be resolved as soon as possible. The right to refuse treatment can be difficult for staff when a patient who has mental capacity refuses a life-saving treatment, but this must be respected. It is a basic principle in law that an adult who is mentally competent has the right to refuse treatment contrary to medical advice (Fig. 10.4).

Whilst it must be presumed that adults have capacity to make decisions, it is assumed in law that children do not. In this situation, parental consent is required, and in law, a child becomes an adult on their 18th birthday. However, just as an adult can be found to be unable to make decisions, a child can be declared able to make best-interest decisions by a health professional in certain situations. As a healthcare professional, you have a duty of care to keep children safe whilst also balancing this with their needs and wishes (NSPCC, 2022). There may be circumstances in which it is appropriate to determine whether they are mature enough to consent for themselves. When assessing a child's

---

What is valid consent?

- The patient must be competent to make a decision
- The patient must have sufficient information to make a decision
- Their decision must be freely given and not under the influence of others or duress

Fig. 10.4   **What is valid consent?**

competence, your supervisor may tell you about Gillick competence or Fraser guidelines. Whilst both terms come from the same legal case in 1985 (Gillick v West Norfolk and Wisbech AHA), they are different. Fraser guidelines (named after Lord Fraser) still relate to the advice and treatment given in relation to contraception and sexual health. Gillick competence is used in a wider context to assess whether a child can make their own choices and understand the consequences of those decisions. It is always recommended that children should be encouraged to share information with their parents or carers about their decision-making and to provide the support to do so. However, when this is not an option for the child, Gillick and Fraser guidelines should be used.

As outlined in the Mental Capacity Act (2005) and Family Reform Act (1969), it can be presumed that 16- and 17-year-olds can be competent and have the capacity to consent to medical treatment. In some circumstances, however, their refusal can be overridden by a parent or the courts, which is not the case for adults (CQC, 2022). This is because of the overriding duty to act in the best interests of a child and would be applicable to a situation in which a refusal would likely lead to death, severe injury or physical or mental harm to the individual. There isn't a lower age limit with regards to Gillick competence or Fraser guidelines. However, it would be seldom safe or correct for a child under 13 to consent to treatment without the knowledge of a parent or carer. Under-13-year-olds cannot consent in law to sexual activity, so regardless of a Gillick competence assessment, this situation would require action, and safeguarding processes would need to be followed. Equally, if there are safeguarding concerns about a child under 18, these should be raised, and the young person should be informed of this action unless doing so creates a significant risk to their safety (CQC, 2022).

Are there situations when consent is not required?

In an emergency situation, it may be difficult to obtain informed consent. Decisions and actions need to be taken quickly, but the principles of consent remain the same. If a person is conscious and has capacity, consent should still be obtained. If consent is not obtained, there must be clear medical reasons as to why it was unsafe to wait to obtain consent. The General Medical Council (2020) explains that:

- If a patient is unconscious or it's not possible to find out their wishes and you have decided they lack capacity, you can provide treatment that is immediately necessary to save their life or to prevent a serious harm.
- If there is more than one option, the care you provide should be the least restrictive of the patient's rights and freedoms, including their future choices.
- For as long as the patient lacks capacity, you should provide ongoing care.
- If the patient regains capacity while in your care, as soon as they are sufficiently recovered to understand, you must tell them what has been done so far and why.

Whilst this guidance was written for doctors, it is also relevant for nurses. The Mental Health Act (1983), which was updated in 2007, is the main legislation for how to assess and treat those with a mental health disorder. It provides instructions for other circumstances where consent is not required. This legislation relates to when the patient has a severe mental health condition, such as bipolar disorder, dementia or schizophrenia, and does not have the capacity to consent to the treatment of their mental health condition. Treating unrelated physical health conditions should still require consent, which the patient, despite their mental health condition, may still be able to give. Equally, the National Assistance Act, 1948, allows for those who are severely ill and living in unsanitary conditions to be taken to a place of care without their consent (NHS, 2022). Furthermore, the Mental Health Act (1983, 2007) legislates that if a patient needs hospital treatment for a severe mental health condition but is refusing treatment and was competent when they attempted suicide or self-harmed, an approved social worker or close relative must make an application for the person to be forcibly kept in hospital, and they must be assessed by two doctors.

When a person is unable to make decisions for themselves and have a say in their care, it is important that they are listened to and that their rights are protected. In 2005, the Mental Capacity Act gave people who lack capacity the statutory right to receive independent advocacy (Speaking Up, 2007). The Care Act (2014) ensures that all eligible service users and carers are offered a Care Act advocacy service by local authorities.

TIP

Useful questions to determine if someone may need an advocacy service. Ask:

- Do they have difficulty understanding relevant information?
- Do they have difficulty retaining information?
- Are they able to weigh up the information (e.g., the pros and cons) to reach a decision?
- Are they able to communicate their wishes, feelings and choices?

Reflect back upon a recent situation in which you observed or contributed to the care of a patient. How was the information communicated to the patient and consent obtained? How was this recorded in their notes and by whom? If you had to recount this scenario in a statement in a courtroom, would you be able to do this? Would the written records 'hold up' in court?

_____

_____

_____

_____

As a nursing student, it is important that you understand the legal and ethical rationale for consent and support your patients to make meaningful decisions. Communicating information clearly is a key responsibility and skill for all nurses. The principles of informed consent should be applied when obtaining consent in order to promote and protect patient autonomy. Your responsibilities also include the requirement to maintain patient confidentiality, which means not disclosing information confided to you by a patient.

CONFIDENTIALITY

This duty arises once the disclosure has been made and is a legal obligation that is derived from case law and within professional codes of conduct, including the NMC code (2018). The requirement to maintain confidentiality as an employee of an NHS trust is found within all contracts of employment and also underpinned by the NHS code of practice on confidentiality (DH, 2003; NHS England and NHS Improvement, 2019). As a nursing student, you are also required to maintain these requirements of confidentiality as part of your scope of practice. This also applies to your academic work, whether it's a tutorial discussion, assessment or essay.

TIP

DO NOT include the names of patients, family members or carers in your academic work.

The only exception to this is the names of individuals that are now cited in the public domain, for example, the Victoria Climbie Inquiry (Laming, 2003). It is expected that these sources are referenced.

DO NOT include any identifiable information or details such as a date of birth, hospital number, copies of care plans and so on that could allow the reader to identify the individual.

DO NOT name organisations, locations and clinical areas which could identify your placement setting to the reader.

DO NOT name individuals you are working with such as healthcare professionals, volunteers, other students or teaching staff.

DO use the name of your workplace and supervisor in your placement documentation, e.g., time sheets. This is necessary to ensure authenticity.

DO reference generic trust documents such as leaflets or policies if they are freely available on the internet for public access and do not identify your placement area. If a local policy would disclose your placement area, use the generic term NHS Trust within the text and again in the reference list with (name withheld) included.

TIP

DO use a pseudonym when including discussion relating to patients, family, carers or colleagues and highlight that you are doing so to your reader.

DO reference appropriate sources which illustrate your requirement to maintain confidentiality, such as the NMC code (2018) or Data Protection Act (2018).

In order for patients to feel able to confide personal information about themselves to nurses, there needs to be trust. The patient needs to be able to trust the nurse or health professional in order to be open and honest and to not refrain from sharing important information that may be essential to their care provision. The NMC code outlines its requirements clearly.

NMC

THE NMC SAYS

'Respect people's right to privacy and confidentiality

As a nurse, midwife, or nursing associate, you owe a duty of confidentiality to all those who are receiving care. This includes making sure that they are informed about their care and that information about them is shared appropriately. To achieve this, you must:

5.1 Respect a person's right to privacy in all aspects of their care

5.2 Make sure that people are informed about how and why information is used and shared by those who will be providing care

5.3 Respect that a person's right to privacy and confidentiality continues after they have died

5.4 Share necessary information with other health and care professionals and agencies only when the interests of patient safety and public protection override the need for confidentiality

5.5 Share with people, their families, and their carers, as far as the law allows, the information they want or need to know about their health, care, and ongoing treatment sensitively and in a way, they can understand'.

It can be argued that with an ever-ageing population how information sharing with families takes place, can be challenging. Whilst information can be shared, it should only be done so once the patient has provided permission, which may be challenging at times. Where a patient cannot receive the information or consent to disclosure, it may be judged to be appropriate to disclose to a relative. Castle (2019) explains that it is important to take the approach that *the diagnosis belongs to the patient and not the relatives*, and this will help avoid the difficult situation in which family members request that a diagnosis is kept from the patient. Castle (2019) goes on to suggest that the concept of confidentiality can be a *minefield for the inexperienced nurse* and recommends suggesting that the patient nominate one family member to be the person with whom information is shared. The rest of the family then goes to the nominated person, who acts as the conduit with the permission of the patient.

Maintaining a patient's confidentiality is a duty fundamental to professional nursing practice, but there are situations in which exceptions arise and information can be disclosed. First and foremost, information can be disclosed with the express permission of whoever originally imparted it. Therefore, if a patient provides permission for you to share information with other health and social care professionals also involved in the care of the patient, this is acceptable. These professionals are also bound by the duty of confidentiality, and this should be explained to the patient when the explicit consent is obtained. This ensures that the patient understands how the information will be used and has no objections. If they do object and won't allow their information to be shared with other healthcare professionals, this can impact the safety and continuity of the care they can be offered, and the patient should be informed of this (Griffith, 2015).

There are also certain situations which allow for disclosure of information without consent (Griffith, 2016) (Fig. 10.5).

Raising concerns and whistle-blowing

Alongside a nurse's duty to obtain consent and maintain confidence is a duty to report incidents and raise concerns. It is understood that in your role as a nurse and whilst you are a nursing student, it is possible that you may come across situations and identify risks that need to be raised with employers or the NMC. Whistle-blowing in healthcare is

In the interests of justice	When it is a matter of public interest or for the public good	In order to protect a third party
There may be a statutory (legal) requirement or court order for the information.	Here the courts must consider two competing interests and weigh up whether it is in the public interest for the information to remain 'secret' or whether it is in the public interest for the information to be shared.	To prevent death or immediate harm, or when there is a safeguarding risk of harm.
e.g., Disclosure of information in order to prevent or detect a serious crime.	e.g., The sharing of information between the police and regulatory bodies such as the NMC in order that investigations can be undertaken.	e.g., When there is a case of suspected abuse of a child or an at-risk adult.

Fig. 10.5   **When disclosure may be acceptable and justifiable by the law.**

when a worker raises a concern about wrongdoing in the public interest (NMC, 2022). Whistle-blowing can be within an organisation, but sometimes, people don't feel able to do this. Therefore, the law recognises a third person, known as a 'prescribed person'. The NMC is named as a prescribed person and has a legal duty to share the information about whistle-blowing reports they have received in an annual report (NMC, 2022). This joint report shows how different agencies work together to tackle serious issues raised with them. The law sets out a clear set of criteria that must be met for the NMC to consider that a whistle-blowing concern has been raised. The types of whistle-blowing concerns that can be raised with the NMC include concerns relating to the education of those wishing to gain pre- or postregistration qualifications and the conduct of nurses, midwives and nursing associates in relation to:

- Their registration or revalidation
- Their fitness to practice
- Noncompliance or concerns about compliance with legislation, policies or standards. (NMC, 2022)

GAINING CONFIDENCE

Being confident about your roles and responsibilities with regard to topics such as consent and confidentiality will enable you to become a competent practitioner and fulfil your duty of care. It is worth taking the time to understand your ethical and legal duties and to consider how you will ensure you remain up to date with your knowledge and practice to ensure that you are always confident with your working practices and doing the best for your patients.

The prospect of potentially having to be a whistle-blower at some point in the future is a daunting one, particularly when you are starting out on your nursing journey. It may feel that there are lots of rules and regulations to follow, and the responsibilities you will hold and how to conduct yourself in a practice setting can be a little overwhelming to begin with. However, in order to protect the public and fulfil your responsibilities as a nursing student and registrant, it is important that you take your duties seriously, including the requirement to raise concerns when necessary. As part of your preparation for practice and your induction process, it is helpful to be aware of how best to raise concerns and what are the appropriate channels of communication to use when you are in practice, learning as a nursing student. Equally, it is useful to become familiar with where to go to for support for all aspects of your training. The importance of reflecting and having professional discussions to develop your learning should not be underestimated.

Data protection

'With the vast majority of personal data breaches being caused by human error, protecting personal information is a team sport with the actions of individuals making a critical difference, good or bad. In the wrong circumstances, the accidental disclosure of something seemingly minor like an address can result in actual physical harm to someone.

In Healthcare settings student nurses will be regularly in contact with sensitive personal data so the application of their university learning and awareness of their data protection responsibilities is essential in protecting patient's rights. They should be unafraid of acting if they see shortcomings as this will be in the best interests of all concerned'.

Matt Robbins, Head of Information Rights, The Open University

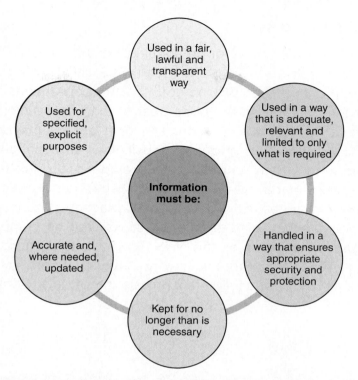

Fig. 10.6   **Data protection principles (RCN, 2023). (The figure was created using the data from RCN (2023) Data protection and monitoring at work. Available at: Data protection and monitoring at work I Advice guides I Royal College of Nursing (rcn.org.uk) (Accessed 19.05.23))**

In 2018, the General Data Protection Regulations (GDPR) came into effect, which govern how personal information is used by businesses, organisations and the government. If you are responsible for using personal data, there are strict principles that you must follow to protect all data and information, whether digital or printed. These are shown in Fig. 10.6. Personal data is defined as any data relating to an identifiable living person. Opinion and facts about people can be defined as personal data if you can identify the person from the context of the information.

It is also useful to be aware that there is stronger legal protection for more sensitive information, including (but not limited to) race, ethnic background, political opinions, religious beliefs, trade union membership, biometrics (where used for identification) and health (RCN, 2023).

Impact of a data breach

The loss, theft or disclosure of personal information is a serious issue which could result in exposure of highly sensitive and confidential information. A data breach will, no doubt, disrupt operations, as well as damage the reputation and public's trust of the organisation affected. In addition to causing a loss of trust, a data breach may also result in financial penalties. Part of our responsibilities as healthcare professionals, working within a healthcare provider's organisation, is to ensure we follow guidance and processes with regards to data to guard against potential breaches. Applying best practice to data protection helps reduce the risk of data breaches. As well as complying with GDPR, organisations such as the NHS also have to demonstrate their compliance. All public authorities have to have a data protection officer and assess risk in terms of high-risk processing of data (Griffith, 2018).

SOCIAL MEDIA
@sa_mom_in_uk

'I think paper handovers are a data leak fine waiting to happen. If we can use ipads for bedside obs surely we can do the same for electronic handover sheets?'

Can you think of examples of when you have used paper or electronic records? What are the pros and cons of each?

_____

_____

_____

_____

TIP

Data: Your rights and responsibilities

- At induction—As part of your placement induction process, you should be shown various policy documents, including the organisation's data protection policy. This outlines the rights and responsibilities of both you and the employer. As a student, the policies also apply to you. Your university will also have a policy and a student privacy notice which set out how your data is used.
- If your data is breached—you should contact the organisation's data protection officer, who will talk you through the process and offer advice regarding next steps. Your tutor should also be made aware so they can support you.
- If you become aware of a data breach involving a patient, you have a professional duty to protect patients from harm, which includes taking action and reporting any concerns.

CASE STUDY

Arjun, a first-year mental health nurse, was on placement at an in-patient setting. He had been working with the nurse in charge, and they were on their way to sit down at the nurses' station when she spotted some visitors who seemed to be filming with their phone. It was the family of a patient, and he was in a six-bedded bay, so there were other patients and families there as well. She approached the person with the phone and asked them if they would stop filming. He said he was making a video for his dad's brother who couldn't visit, as he lived too far away. The nurse explained that the filming could not take place on the ward because of other patients in the room who were in the background. Arjun learned that this was a breach of confidentiality, as you can't film other patients without their consent. At first, the visitor tried to ask permission from the other patients, but the nurse told him that this was not appropriate, as they were unwell (and one was asleep!). The family accepted this, and the son stopped filming. He said they would make a call instead, and he apologised, saying he hadn't realised.

Continued

CASE STUDY—cont'd

Arjun was impressed with the way the nurse handled the situation. He felt that if she had approached it differently, it might have turned into an argument, but in his reflection, which he wrote up the next day, he wrote that she was professional and polite but very clear about her responsibilities to the patients. Arjun was glad to be working with the nurse in charge that shift, as he didn't think he could have had that conversation with the visitor on his first placement. It made him think about the use of phones and how they are everywhere now. Chances are, Arjun added to his reflection, we're all in the background of someone's video or photo. However, this incident helped him learn that it is different in healthcare when we are looking after patients. Arjun was also reminded that nursing students have to think about their responsibilities and remember the NMC code (2018) so that they can protect the safety of their patients and speak up on their behalf.

SOCIAL MEDIA
@JakeUKRN

'Dear nurses, taking a shortcut is the quickest way to commit mistakes. The busier the shift gets, the more imperative it is to follow protocols. They are there to protect everyone. #nhsnurse#safenursingpractice'

CONCLUSION

In this chapter, you have had the opportunity to consider the knowledge, skills and behaviours needed in your student placements and future nursing practice to deliver safe and effective care. The safety of your patient should be your priority, and important aspects of practice have been examined, such as record-keeping, consent and confidentiality. These must be demonstrated and developed throughout your training programme and, once qualified, at revalidation. It is also clear that familiarity with the NMC's code (2018b) is required beyond the classroom and whilst in practice so that you understand your legal responsibilities and can apply this learning to your delivery of care. Being a nurse involves a legal duty of care, and it is essential as a student and future nurse to understand the legal and ethical rationale to inform your decision-making and to justify your actions. This will ensure that you are able to meet all of the code's requirements to practice effectively and prioritise the safety and care of your patients. In turn, this will promote trust for you and the nursing profession.

Now you have finished this chapter. Please make notes on what you have learned.

_____

_____

_____

_____

_____

_____

_____

_____

_____

_____

_____

_____

_____

_____

_____

_____

_____

_____

REFERENCES

Avery, G. (2013) *Law and Ethics in Nursing and Healthcare: An Introduction.* London, Sage Publications Ltd.

Andrews, A. and St. Aubyn, B. (2015) 'If it's not written down; it didn't happen'. *Journal of Community Nursing*, 2015, 29(5), pp. 20–22.

Care Act 2014, c.23. Available at: http://www.legislation.gov.uk/ukpga/2014/23/contents/enacted (Accessed: 29 May 2023).

Castle, N. (2019) 'A matter of confidentiality'. *British Journal of Nursing* Vol 28, No 4, p. 218. DOI: 10.12968/bjon.2019.28.4.218

CQC (2022) *GP mythbuster 8: Gillick competency and Fraser guidelines.* Available at: GP mythbuster 8: Gillick competency and Fraser guidelines - Care Quality Commission (cqc.org.uk) (Accessed 09.06.23)

Data Protection Act (2018) Available at: Data Protection Act 2018 (legislation.gov.uk) (Accessed 09.06.23)

Dimond, B. (2011) *Legal Aspects of Nursing.* 6th edition. Harlow, Pearson Education Limited.

DH (2003) 'Confidentiality: NHS Code of Practice'. Available at: 78051-DoH-NHS Code-Practice (publishing.service.gov.uk) (Accessed: 26 June 2023).

Embury-Dennis, T. (2018) 'NHS workers disciplined for accessing Ed Sheeran's health records' *The Independent.* Saturday 18th May. Available at: NHS workers disciplined 'for accessing Ed Sheeran's health records' | The Independent | The Independent (Accessed: 18 May 2023).

Family Reform Act (1969) Available at: Family Law Reform Act 1969 (legislation.gov.uk) (Accessed: 9 June 2023).

General Medical Council (2020) *Circumstances that effect the decision-making process: Treatment in emergencies.* Available at Circumstances that affect the decision-making process part one of four - ethical guidance - GMC (gmc-uk.org) (Accessed: 26 May 2023).

Gillick v West Norfolk and Wisbeck Area Health Authority [1985] 3 All ER 402 [1986] AC 112 HL

Griffith, R. (2016) 'For the record: Keeping detailed notes'. *British Journal of Nursing,* 25(7), pp. 408–409. DOI: 10.12968/bjon.2016.25.7.408

Griffith, R. (2018) 'District nurses must guard against inappropriately accessing patient records'. *British Journal of Community Nursing*, 23(7), pp. 355–357. DOI: 10.12968/bjcn.2018.23.7.355

Griffith, R. (2015) 'Understanding the code: Exceptions to the duty of confidentiality'. *British Journal of Community Nursing*, 20(7), pp. 356–359. DOI: 10.12968/bjcn.2015.20.7.356

Laming, L. (2003). The Victoria Climbié inquiry: report of an inquiry by Lord Laming. London: The Stationery Office. Available at The Victoria Climbie Inquiry: report of an inquiry by Lord Laming - GOV.UK (www.gov.uk) (Accessed: 11 June 2023).

Mental Capacity Act (2005) Available at: Mental Capacity Act 2005 (legislation.gov.uk) (Accessed: 9 June 2023).

Mental Health Act (1983) Available at: Mental Health Act 1983 (legislation.gov.uk) (Accessed: 26 May 2023).

Mental Health Act (2007) Available at: Mental Health Act 2007 (legislation.gov.uk) (Accessed: 26 May 2023).

NHS England (2017) 'Involving people in their own health and care: statutory guidance for clinical commissioning groups and NHS England'. Available at NHS England " Involving people in their own health and care: statutory guidance for clinical commissioning groups and NHS England (Accessed: 18 May 2023).

NHS England and NHS Improvement (2019) Confidentiality policy. Available at: NHS England report template - data icon (Accessed: 26 May 2023).

NHS Professionals (2018) 'Delegating record keeping and countersigning records: Guidance for nursing staff' *Quality Matters*, Issue 06. Available at 9179CBA2A55D40E9A9D-E3B665B6A5A47.ashx (nhsprofessionals.nhs.uk) (Accessed: 17 May 2023).

NMC (2018a) *Future nurse: Standards of proficiency for registered nurses.* Available at: future-nurse-proficiencies.pdf (nmc.org.uk) (Accessed: 16 May 2023).

NMC Code (2018b) *The code: Professional standards of practice and behaviour for nurses, midwives and nursing associates.* London: Nursing and Midwifery Council [Available from: https://www.nmc.org.uk/globalassets/sitedocuments/nmc-publications/nmc-code.pdf (Accessed: 17 May 2023).

NMC (2019) *What must be in place.* Available at: What must be in place - The Nursing and Midwifery Council (nmc.org.uk) (Accessed: 9 June 2023).

NMC (2020) *Fitness to practise committee substantive order review hearing*, 14 Feb 2020. Available at: reasons-aram-ftpcsorh-65112-20200214.pdf (nmc.org.uk)- (Accessed: 9 June 2023).

NMC (2023a) *Revalidation.* Available at: Revalidation - The Nursing and Midwifery Council (nmc.org.uk) (Accessed: 16 May 2023).

NMC (2023b) *Fitness to practise committee substantive order review hearing*, 29 July 2022. Available at: reasons-morris-ftpcsm-76986-20220729.pdf (nmc.org.uk) (Accessed: 9 June 2023).

NMC (2023c) *Fitness to practise committee substantive order review hearing*, 27-30 June 2022 reasons-stephen-ftpcsh-74379-20220630.pdf (nmc.org.uk) (Accessed: 9 June 2023).

NMC (2023d) *Professionalism.* Available at: Professionalism - The Nursing and Midwifery Council (nmc.org.uk) (Accessed: 7 July 2023).

NMC (2022) Whistleblowing to the NMC: What is whistleblowing? Available at: Whistleblowing to the NMC - The Nursing and Midwifery Council (Accessed: 26 May 2023).

NSPCC (2022) *Gillick competency and Fraser guidelines.* Available at: Gillick competence and Fraser guidelines I NSPCC Learning (Accessed: 22 May 2023).

Peate, I. (2017). 'Chapter 5: Duty of care' *Fundamentals of Care: A Textbook for Health and Social Care Assistants*, John Wiley & Sons, Incorporated. ProQuest Ebook Central. P57 Available at: ProQuest Ebook Central - Book Details (Accessed: 7 July 2023).

RCN (2023) *Data protection and monitoring at work.* Available at: Data protection and monitoring at work I Advice guides I Royal College of Nursing (rcn.org.uk) (Accessed: 19 May 2023).

Smith, M. (2016) 'Nurse sacked after inappropriately accessing patients' hospital records' *Wales Online*. Available at: Nurse sacked after 'inappropriately' accessing patients' hospital records - Wales Online (Accessed: 19 May 2023).

Speaking Up (2007) *Making decisions: The Independent Mental Capacity Advocate (IMCA) Service* OPG606. Available at: Making decisions. The Independent Mental Capacity Advocate (IMCA) service (publishing.service.gov.uk) (Accessed 09.06.23)

Stevens, S. and Pickering, D. (2010) 'Keeping good records: A guide'. *Community Eye Health,* 23(74), p. 44-45. ISSN: 0953-6833

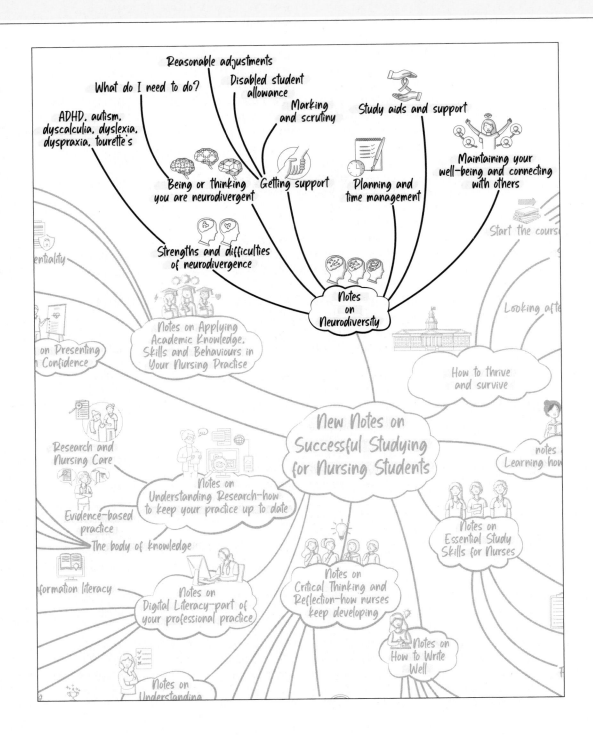

NOTES ON NEURODIVERSITY

Rachael Major (she/her)

INTRODUCTION

It is important to understand what neurodiversity is and the challenges and benefits that it can bring for a nursing student. This chapter will discuss how to identify if you might be neurodivergent, what support and reasonable adjustments you might be able to access and study skills and tips for practice. It will also address maintaining your well-being as a neurodivergent student.

Neurodiversity was a term first coined in the late 1990s by Judy Singer, an Australian sociology student at the time. Neurodiversity describes the range of differences in the way people think, act, move and understand the world around us. It recognises that differences are important and bring benefits to society. In short, we are all neurodiverse. However, for some, their strengths and challenges lay outside society norms (being 'neurotypical'), and this is neurodivergence. However, neurodiversity has also been used as a term to describe a group of conditions that are associated with neurodivergence, commonly autism, attention deficit hyperactivity disorder (ADHD), dyslexia, dyspraxia (also known as developmental coordination disorder), dyscalculia and Tourette's syndrome, although this is not an exhaustive list.

It is thought that 15%–20% of the population is neurodivergent (Neurodiversity Celebration Week, 2023), although, in my experience, this is much higher in nursing students. In several of my student nursing groups, more than half are neurodivergent. There may be many reasons for this, but it could be that neurodivergent people are attracted to certain professions and ways of working.

The next section of this chapter will describe the common difficulties that nursing can pose to people with different conditions associated with neurodivergence, as well as their strengths. Neurodivergent people may find some things really difficult and other things incredibly easy. The following gives a very general overview of strengths and challenges associated with the different conditions, but these are, by necessity, generalisations and overly simplistic, as everyone is an individual who will experience different challenges in different contexts. Areas of strengths and difficulties associated with these different conditions overlap, and it is common to have more than one condition.

STRENGTHS AND DIFFICULTIES ASSOCIATED WITH NEURODIVERGENCE

Attention deficit hyperactivity disorder

Approximately 5% of children and 3.5% of adults in the United Kingdom have been diagnosed with the neurodevelopmental condition ADHD (NICE, 2022), although this is likely to be a low estimate. ADHD starts in childhood and presents in different ways in different people, but there are inattentive forms where children struggle to focus, are easily distracted, don't seem to listen and are disorganised, and the hyperactive/impulsive forms where children fidget, are always on the go, interrupt, are excessively talkative and do not think before they engage in potentially risky behaviour. It is possible to have a combined type of ADHD where children have all or most of these behaviours. It used to be thought that children grew out of ADHD, but we now recognise that this is not always the case and that symptoms in adulthood can be different. For example, hyperactivity is more likely to be a feeling of inner restlessness, and adults develop strategies to overcome or compensate for some of their difficulties. We also know that both children and adults can hyperfocus on activities that they find stimulating, although this can

TABLE 11.1 STRENGTHS AND CHALLENGES ASSOCIATED WITH ADHD

Strengths associated with ADHD	Challenges of ADHD
• Can hyperfocus on tasks and be extremely productive • Creative and entrepreneurial • Can view things from different perspectives • Problem-solving skills • Empathy • Energetic • Enthusiastic • Hard working • Interested in new things • Sensitive	• Poor attention or attention to detail • Hyperactivity or restlessness (might be an inner restlessness or feeling of always needing to be doing something) • Poor time management, sense of time/prioritisation • Impulsiveness • Overworking, difficulty relaxing • Forgetfulness • Excessive talking or talking over people • Sensitive to rejection

cause challenges, for example, spending hours on computer games (Table 11.1).

Autism

Autism is a spectrum condition, which means that it affects people differently and is lifelong. Autistic people see the world differently, and this can affect the way that they interact with others and their environment and their interests. Sensory sensitivities are common for autistic people, meaning that certain lights, sounds, smells, touch, tastes and textures can be difficult, even potentially physically painful. For others, they may seek sensory experiences, and senses can get muddled, such as seeing sounds and smelling colours (synaesthesia) (Table 11.2).

Women and girls with ADHD and autism

Women and girls with ADHD and autism can present differently to men and boys and therefore are less likely to be diagnosed earlier in life.

TABLE 11.2 STRENGTHS AND CHALLENGES ASSOCIATED WITH AUTISM

Strengths associated with autism	Challenges of autism
• Attention to detail • Good at following and developing protocols and procedures • Can view things from different perspectives • Problem-solving skills • Efficient • Logical • Retain knowledge • Focus	• Difficulty interpreting verbal and nonverbal language, e.g., facial expression, tone of voice • Literal understanding of language • Difficulty reading the subtleties of neurotypical people • Sensory sensitivities • Repetitive or routine behaviours • Meltdowns or shutdowns

Girls with ADHD tend to show less hyperactivity and impulsivity than boys and are more likely to be inattentive, although this is not always the case. Girls tend to have better social skills and may learn to 'fit in' better, are less disruptive in school and may get into trouble less. The media often also depict ADHD and autism as being conditions associated with white boys or men—think of films such as *Forest Gump* and *Rain Man* or TV dramas. Girls with autism and ADHD can therefore fall under the radar and be misunderstood. They are more likely to be diagnosed with anxiety, depression or other mental health conditions such as personality disorders.

Dyscalculia

Dyscalculia is a learning difference that affects mathematical skills. It does not mean that you cannot ever do maths, but it does mean that you find it harder to grasp mathematical concepts and learn mathematical facts and sequences and that maths doesn't come naturally. Your maths abilities are not consistent with your age, educational opportunities or your intellectual abilities. Even if you get the correct answer and use a suitable method, you may lack confidence and may not know why you have got to that answer (Table 11.3).

TABLE 11.3 STRENGTHS AND CHALLENGES ASSOCIATED WITH DYSCALCULIA

Strengths associated with dyscalculia	Challenges of dyscalculia
• Problem-solving skills • Different ways of looking at things • Creativity • Strategic thinking • Empathy • Good with words • Socially skilled	• Difficulty understanding numbers • Poor sense of understanding of numbers • Slow to perform calculations • Difficulty remembering maths formulas and facts • Difficulty counting backward • Difficulty remembering sequences • Difficulties with time management and reading time

Dyslexia

Dyslexia is a learning difference that primarily affects the ability to read fluently and accurately and spelling (Rose, 2009), although, for some, it can also cause difficulties in processing both visual and auditory information (British Dyslexia Association, 2010). People with dyslexia often find that they have to reread information a number of times before they can fully understand it, and this means that reading can be slower, especially when you have to read a lot of complex texts. Visual stress (also known as stereoscopic sensitivity or Meares-Irlen syndrome) is a separate condition where the words or letters may move around the page or the page seems excessively bright, making reading very uncomfortable. This can be helped with coloured lenses or overlays (Table 11.4).

Dyspraxia (or developmental coordination disorder)

Dyspraxia is a condition that affects motor coordination, which is thought to affect about 6% of children and often co-occurs with other neurodevelopmental conditions (Lino and Chieffo, 2022) (Table 11.5).

TABLE 11.4 STRENGTHS AND CHALLENGES ASSOCIATED WITH DYSLEXIA

Strengths associated with dyslexia	Challenges of dyslexia
• Good at visual and pattern recognition • Innovative • Strong verbal communication skills • Entrepreneurial thinking • See the bigger picture • Creativity • Empathy	• Difficulties with spelling and fluent word reading • Slower verbal processing speed, i.e., taking time to process what is being said • Slower reading • Reduced verbal memory and working memory

TABLE 11.5 STRENGTHS AND CHALLENGES ASSOCIATED WITH DYSPRAXIA

Strengths associated with dyspraxia	Challenges of dyspraxia
• Determination • Hard working • Problem-solving • Creative • Original thinking	• Poor motor control/coordination • Clumsiness • Poor time management/ organisation • Difficulty finding the right words • Difficulties with knowing your left and right • Poor spatial awareness

Tourette's syndrome

Tourette's syndrome is a neurodevelopmental condition which is characterised by involuntary movements or sounds called tics. Tics can be simple such as blinking, shoulder shrugging, limb or head jerking, abdominal tensing, sniffing, coughing, grunting or throat clearing, or complex such as twirling, jumping, touching objects or people or uttering words or phrases. Tics involving swearing (or coprolalia) only occur

TABLE 11.6 STRENGTHS AND CHALLENGES ASSOCIATED WITH TOURETTE

Strengths associated with Tourette syndrome	Challenges of Tourette
• Hyperfocus • Interpersonal awareness • Planning ahead • Creativity • Verbal processing • Information processing	• Involuntary movements • Involuntary sounds or words • Embarrassment • Other people's reactions • Worse when stressed, tired or anxious

in 10%–20% of people with Tourette. Tics normally appear in childhood, and for some, they are gone by adulthood; however, this is not the case for all. Some people can suppress tics for a brief time, and some tics are more internal and cannot be seen but can be felt. Stress, tiredness, anxiety, caffeine and bright or flashing lights can make the tics worse (Table 11.6).

Myth busting

- You cannot be a nurse if you are neurodivergent—**Wrong**, there are very many successful neurodivergent nurses working in all areas of nursing. Some of your lecturers may well be neurodivergent, along with senior staff in your practice placements. For example, the chief nursing officer for England, Ruth May, has dyslexia (Matthews et al., 2019).
- Neurodivergent people lack empathy—**Wrong,** neurodivergent people are often very empathetic, and this can be a strength.

SOCIAL MEDIA
@Leia_ND_STN

'I have a lot of empathy (sometimes too much) and am a fierce advocate for people I am caring for due to this'

BEING OR THINKING YOU ARE NEURODIVERGENT _

There are neurodivergent people in all parts of society and from all countries of the world and are not limited to a specific gender, class, skin colour, ethnicity, age or sexuality. The experiences of neurodivergent people will also be influenced by intersectionality, which can affect how neurodivergence is identified and experienced. This can affect mental health and well-being both in childhood and as adults.

I already know that I am neurodivergent

That is good news. If you haven't already made contact with the disability or inclusion team at university, then do this now. They get very busy at the beginning of the academic year, so get in as soon as you can. You may not think that you have a disability and that the service is not for you, or you may feel concerned that disclosing might put you at a disadvantage. Please don't worry; they are very used to supporting neurodivergent students and will let you know what support you can have, even if you don't feel that you need it at the moment. It is better to know what help is available early rather than to try and find out when you are stressed and struggling. If you don't need any help later, then the time is not wasted; you may be able to help a friend or colleague.

I think I might be neurodivergent

It is not uncommon for students to go through the whole of their schooling to then find out that they are neurodivergent at university. This could be for many reasons. The work is harder than at school, you are required to be more self-sufficient, there is a different way of working that you are not used to and you will have to manage placements and study, perhaps whilst living away from home for the first time. You may have had help from family and friends in the past, and they are no longer there to support you as much, or you want to become more independent. All of these things can be challenging for any student. You will have developed strategies to complete your qualifications to get onto your programme, and some of these may not be as effective anymore. We also know that stress can interfere with these strategies, as well as working memory (which is why some of you may not do your best in exams). Your tutor may have suggested that you may have dyslexia, or you may just be reading through this chapter thinking, that's me! If this is the case, contact your university disability or inclusion team, and they can offer support and screening and signpost you to what to do next. If you are not sure, there are a number of online screening tools that you can access, some for free, that you can take before approaching the disability team. These are not diagnostic tools but can be a guide. If you decide to complete one or more of these and they do not identify that you are neurodivergent, but you still think you might be, still contact the team for support.

A warning here, though; it can take time to get a diagnosis, and unfortunately, waiting lists and access to diagnostic assessments vary across the country, especially for autism and ADHD. To be eligible to obtain Disabled Student Allowance (DSA), you need to have evidence of a disability or learning difference from a medical professional or a diagnostic assessment from a suitably qualified psychologist or a specialist teacher with an Assessment Practising Certificate (APC). The disability team will also use these reports to guide your reasonable adjustments. Even if you don't go down the route of getting an 'official diagnosis', many of the tips in this chapter and the rest of the book will still be helpful.

SOCIAL MEDIA
@jade_w08

'Understanding your diagnosis is important for your development, and don't feel bad if a tool does not work for you. You may need time to figure out what works for you and that's fine'.

What actions do you plan to take having read this first part of the chapter?

_____

_____

_____

_____

SUPPORT

What support might I be offered?

Each university has their own system, but here are some areas of support that are generally offered:

- Advice and support with reasonable adjustments both in class and in practice
- Support with claiming DSA
- Exam adjustments
- Assistive technology
- One-on-one support
  - This may include helping to structure assignments
  - Breaking down assignment tasks
  - Ensuring that you have addressed the assignment task
  - Proofreading
  - Planning and time management
  - General study skills

What are reasonable adjustments?

Reasonable adjustments are changes that can be made to reduce any disadvantage that you might have because of your neurodiversity and are defined in the Equality Act (2010) for England, Scotland and Wales or the Disability Discrimination Act (1995) in Northern Ireland. Reasonable adjustments are personal to you and will be decided based on a needs assessment and university regulations; however, they may include:

- Extra time for exams
- Rest breaks in exams
- Access to and use of assistive technology
- A reader or scribe in exams (not in practice)
- A mentor
- Extra time/late submissions for assignments
- Alternative forms of assessment
- Adjustments to practice hours
- Adjustment to practice experiences
- Quiet areas to write notes

It must be remembered that you still need to be able to meet all the requirements of your programme and the Nursing and Midwifery Council (NMC) standards (2018a). This means that you must complete all the 2300 hours of theory and 2300 hours of practice and achieve all the proficiencies. Reasonable adjustments must also be practical; it would not be reasonable to have a scribe in practice, for example.

What is Disabled Student Allowance, and how can it help?

DSA is a fund to help you with your studies which you can apply for if your disability has a 'substantial' impact on your ability to study. This might mean that it takes you longer to read than others in your group or you need additional support to keep on track with your work because of your neurodivergence. DSA is not means tested and may give you money to buy equipment or software to help you with your course or fund additional study support or a mentor, for example. A needs assessment will help decide what will help you best.

To be eligible for DSA, you need to meet several criteria:

- Be an undergraduate or postgraduate student
- Be eligible for student finance
- Be studying a course that lasts for at least a year
- Have evidence that you have a disability
    - For dyslexia, that will be an up-to-date 'diagnostic assessment' from an educational psychologist or specialist dyslexia teacher with an APC
    - For other disabilities, this may be a letter from a doctor or psychiatrist or a completed disability evidence form (see the following websites)

Each country in the United Kingdom has different ways of managing DSA, so you need to ensure that you apply through the most appropriate website. Please see the disability advisors at your university for help with this.

- England: https://www.gov.uk/disabled-students-allowance-dsa
- Wales: https://www.studentfinancewales.co.uk/

- Scotland: https://www.saas.gov.uk/guides/dsa
- Northern Ireland: please see a disability advisor at the university for help rather than apply through DSA online

If you are doing a degree apprenticeship, then you are not able to claim DSA but may be entitled to Access to Work (https://www.gov.uk/access-to-work) through your employer. Once you are registered, you may be entitled to Access to Work, as well as reasonable adjustments from your employer (Equality Act, 2010).

Do I tell anyone I am or think I am neurodivergent?

You will all come into your nursing degree with different experiences of education, and not all of them are likely to be positive. You may be worried what people might think about you and that they may judge you based on poor understanding of neurodiversity. Disclosing or declaring your neurodivergence is your choice, but there are a number of reasons why you might want to:

First, you cannot access reasonable adjustments unless someone is aware or should reasonably be aware that you have a disability. Your nursing programme is hard enough without accessing the support that you are entitled to. You don't need to prove to anyone, least of all yourself, that you can do this without a bit of help. You need to be the most safe and effective nurse that you can be, and this may require reasonable adjustments.

Second, masking (where you try to appear different from your normal self in social situations) is exhausting and does not do your long-term physical or mental health any good at all.

SOCIAL MEDIA
@Leia_ND_STN

'I find it easier to be open about my ASD than to hide it. Most people have been great about it and those who haven't just needed some education or simply aren't worth your time'

It is common for students to tell the university that they are neurodivergent but are more reluctant to do so in practice. Remember that neurodivergence is common, and it is likely that some of your group, lecturers and practice assessors are also neurodivergent, and there is a growing understanding of neurodiversity within the profession. Seek the support of your academic assessor, link tutor or disability advisor if you are concerned about reasonable adjustments or support in practice. You still have to achieve all of your proficiencies to complete your programme (NMC, 2018a) and adhere to the NMC (2018b) code, but reasonable adjustments can help with this.

NMC

THE NMC SAYS

16.3 'Tell someone in authority at the first reasonable opportunity if you experience problems that may prevent you working within the Code or other national standards, taking prompt action to tackle the causes of concern if you can'.

13.4 'Take account of your own personal safety as well as the safety of people in your care'.

CASE STUDY

Although I struggled in school and my parents tried hard to get me support, it wasn't until I went on to do my international hospitality management honours degree that I was formally diagnosed with dyslexia, dyscalculia and dyspraxia. It was the first time I felt education had recognised my difficulties. I then went on to do a master's degree in digital marketing at the same university and then onto a nursing degree.

In my third year of my nursing degree, I was diagnosed with ADHD. I think I must have masked quite a lot prior to that, but since my diagnosis I don't mask as much, as I feel like it's more acceptable for me to just be myself because this is who I am.

Before I started my first university course, I reached out to the inclusion team at my university to inform them of that I had previously been informally diagnosed with dyscalculia and dyslexia at school. The inclusion team organised for a formal psychological assessment to be carried out, free of charge, which is when I was officially diagnosed, and an official evidence-based report supported

Continued

CASE STUDY—cont'd

my reasonable adjustments for learning. I went down the private route when being assessed for ADHD.

When I started my nursing degree, I also met with an inclusion champion within the nursing school, who helped me identify what support I might need for going into placement. These reasonable adjustments are sent to my placement area prior to me starting my placement. I also always have a calculator and notebook in my tunic pocket so I can write notes, I don't forget information and to help me with drug calculations.

I have received DSA during all my university courses. I have been funded for a laptop with resources on it like Read and Write Gold, which helps me with spelling and grammar, and I was provided with recording equipment, which helps me with my slow processing and my memory. I also have Dragon, a speech-to-text app, but I think the read-aloud function is probably the best thing that I use. I also received a printer, and I am funded for ink and paper on a yearly basis. I must print everything to process written information, and I use highlighters over all my documents. DSA also funds proofreading for me, which is extremely supportive. Importantly, we have a study skills department in our university which is open to all students, so it is inclusive for everybody, and they taught me how to write academically. My reasonable adjustments include extra time in exams and the use of a calculator.

I've always known that I'm different. I've always been perceived differently by people everywhere I have gone, and I have experienced unconscious bias and indeed conscious bias throughout my whole life. I was bullied at school for being different. The diagnosis of ADHD was not a surprise to me, as I already had diagnosed neurodivergences and I connected with a lot of the characteristics that I had read about ADHD. This diagnosis has provided me with answers about myself. Being diagnosed has enabled me to get the support that I need to be at the same stage as everybody else. I guess the word equity is right; I don't get extra time just for the sake of it. I'd far rather not have additional support and

CASE STUDY—cont'd

be able to do what others can, but I need the support to be at the same level as everyone else, and I am not ashamed of that. The diagnoses have enabled me to receive the support that I need to manage and be successful. We all learn in different ways and paces.

When I was in high school, I was handed a college perspective in fifth year and told to leave because they didn't think I would be able to go to university or do very much in life. This reaction had a huge impact on my confidence and led to imposter syndrome; however, with the incredible support of my family, I have achieved an honours degree and a master's degree, and I'm now doing a nursing degree. I aspire to do even further higher education in the future and make a difference in the world. I feel like I've proven quite a lot of people wrong; just because you have a learning difficulty does not mean that you cannot achieve! There are so many neurodivergent people who have gone on to achieve so many amazing things in life! I think a lot of neurodivergent people are extremely empathetic, which is the most important attribute in nursing. I believe that my neurodivergences are my superpowers and the experiences that I have had as a neurodivergent have moulded who I am and the things I have achieved in my life so far.

Chloe Jackson, third-year nursing student

Founder of the Support and Understanding for Neurodivergent Nurses (SUNN) project

GAINING CONFIDENCE

So, you have identified that you are neurodivergent; what can you do to help overcome some of the challenges that you might face at university? Lots of what has been written in previous chapters will also help you, so some of this section will signpost you back to them. Here are a few suggestions that might help you to gain higher grades with less stress.

Understand the way that you work best

This is called metacognition, and everybody works differently. You may already know what works best for you, or you might still be finding out. Accessing study skills support will help you with this.

If you work better in the morning, do the more difficult things then and then work on the easier activities later. If you are struggling to get anything done, try an easy win first and then go back to the harder task; you should find it easier once you have started something. If you still have writer's block, write anything; about your topic would be better, but anything will do, as it gets you into the habit of writing.

Consider also how you learn and use this to help you. Do you learn better by doing things? If so, try to get as involved with the work as much as possible: make things, engage in learning through virtual reality or interactive resources or practice skills and relate this to the theory that you have learnt. If you learn more visually, consider watching videos or making posters or infographics. For those who like to listen, try podcasts or listening back to lectures. Many people like a combination of approaches, so find what works best for you, and use the guidance in the earlier chapters to help. See Chapter 2 for further information about metacognition.

Planning and time management

Unfortunately, there is no getting away from it; it is going to take some of you longer than your peers to do the work, and you will have to work harder than them to get there. It is very frustrating to see some of your peers doing what seems like little work and getting great grades when you cannot do that. Leaving things to the last minute is never a good idea, especially if you find it takes you longer to read and write assignments or are the king or queen of procrastination. At the beginning of the year, know when the assignments are due and use a study planner and/or a diary to organise yourself. Don't forget to plan in time to get study support and to have downtime. Wall planners are good as visual reminders, but these can be used with both paper and electronic diaries and to-do lists. See Chapter 2 for other information about planning and time management that you might find useful.

Use of colour coding and highlighting

Many students have told me that they find colour coding helpful with both learning and organising their work. This can involve different-coloured folders for different topics or the use of different-coloured pens within your notes. For example, you could use a different colour for a section that you feel that you need to go back and learn more on or you are not clear about so that it stands out for you and you don't have to hunt for it in your notes later, or another colour for a topic that you think might be relevant for an assignment coming up or useful in practice. Find what works for you, and don't go over the top with the colours; otherwise, it can be overwhelming or just confusing.

The use of highlighters can also be useful when reading to pick out key information for use in assignments. You can do this on paper or use the tools in Read & Write Gold, ClaroRead, OneNote, Adobe and Kindle, for example. Use the colour coding as above; otherwise, highlighting may not be the most effective use of your time (see Chapter 2).

Make use of study support

If you receive DSA, you may be entitled to additional study support, either through the university or through external organisations; make the best use of this. Seek the support of your tutors. Make sure that you fully understand the assignment task and plan it out. Give yourself plenty of time, especially if you take longer to read and/or write. Earlier chapters of this book will help you with study skills.

Don't ever be embarrassed or afraid of submitting a draft if you are entitled to do so, whatever state you think it is in. Tutors would much rather support you to put things right before you submit the final version than to have to support you through a resubmission.

SOCIAL MEDIA
@Leia_ND_STN

'Don't be afraid to ask questions and ask for clarification, I find it easier to understand information if I know the rationale behind it. Make use of tutorials and 1:1 time with tutors, advocate for yourself when it comes to reasonable adjustments, know when you're near burnout'

Use assistive technology

There are lots of tools that can help you both for studying and in practice. Microsoft (2023), Apple and Google are all incorporating assistive technology more into their systems, and there is specialist software that you might be given as part of DSA or may be available from your university, but here are a few tips that will help:

TIP

- You should be offered training in the use of any assistive technology that you receive from DSA; make the most of this.
- Use text-to-speech to read out your work—it will help with proofreading—and read what you have written rather than what you think you have written, which might not be the same. Examples include Naturally Speaking, Read & Write Gold, ClaroRead and Read Aloud in Word. There are also scanning pens that you can get to read from books, or take photos and use software, such as Naturally Speaking, Office Lens or Speechify, to read it out for you.
- Use grammar support software such as Grammarly or tools already included in your word-processing software.
- Speech-to-text software will help you to put words on paper. This can be particularly helpful if you want to get thoughts out of your head while you remember them, you think faster than you can write or type or your own writing is illegible when you go back to it later, and it can be good for making notes. Examples include

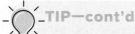

TIP—cont'd

Dragon, Siri and Otter.ai, and it is built-in in newer versions of Google and Microsoft software.

- Mind-mapping software can be helpful to plan out your thoughts. Some people find it difficult to get from a mind map to an organised plan or piece of work, and this is where additional study skills support can help. Examples include MindView, Xmind and Scapple.
- Adobe Acrobat Reader can read out PDF files.
- Access the class presentation before the session. This will allow you to write notes on them or just listen and not have to take notes. Some students may have access to a notetaker for class as part of DSA. Examples include Notably, One Note, Evernote and Google Keep.
- You may be able to record lectures, or they might be recorded for you (check with your university and ask permission of lecturers). Listen back to them to reinforce and check your understanding.
- Take photographs and then add them into software such as OneNote, which will allow you to add notes or speech from lectures into text.
- For those with visual stress (Meares-Irlen syndrome), changing the background colour on a document may help. You can do this in Word and Google Docs. Read & Write Gold and ClaroRead have this included in the package.
- There is also a lot of software that help with reminders. Examples include Alexa, phones, Remember the Milk, Microsoft To Do and Google Keep.
- The website Diversity and Ability has collated both free and paid resources, which may be useful, at https://diversityandability.com/resources/.

Avoid distractions

Avoiding distractions can be particularly difficult for those with ADHD, as everything can be potentially distracting. Some people like complete silence; others need some background noise. Noise-cancelling headphones may help some, especially if you are working in a shared room or the library. If you like a bit of background noise, try white or brown noise or classical music, especially if you are prone to singing along to your favourite tune. Try to keep your desk or workspace as clear as possible, as this has been proven to help make you more productive and make sure that you have everything you need when you start.

Use an app such as Forest (https://www.forestapp.cc) to prevent you from using your phone or another device when you should be studying. Forest uses the Pomodoro technique and asks you to plant trees which will then die if you use your phone or device in the time that you are studying. At the end of your study session, you can see how many trees you have planted, thus giving a reward.

The Pomodoro technique is based around a time management technique where you work for 25 minutes followed by a 5-minute break, which you do for four sessions and then have a 15-minute break. If you are unable to concentrate for 25 minutes, try to work for a shorter period of time and then build that time up as you get into the flow (please see Chapter 2 for further information).

Body doubling

Working with someone can be useful for some, especially if you are prone to procrastination or find getting started with your work difficult. You don't have to be physically with the person; you can work with someone online through a virtual chat or through systems such as Microsoft Teams or Zoom. Focusmate is another tool that you can use for this, where you book a session with someone else online and share your goals. This helps to hold you accountable for making some progress and can increase productivity (Focusmate, 2023).

Practice placements

Neurodivergent nursing students have additional pressures that other students and even neurodivergent registered nurses often don't have. Students are required to continually change placements, and this means that they work in different environments and with different staff. There will be placements that play to your strengths and others which you will find more challenging, but all need to be passed. Once you are registered, it is likely that you will look to work in an area that suits you. You will also develop strategies to help work around areas that you find more difficult whilst maintaining safe and effective nursing practice (Royal College of Nursing, no date).

TIP

As a student, here are some things that might help you:

- Speak to your practice assessor and practice supervisors at the start of the placement about any reasonable adjustments you have and how you learn best. Don't forget to discuss your strengths, too. For example, does it take you a bit longer to learn something new, but once you have got it, you are great at it?
- After handover, check your understanding with your practice supervisor/assessor and plan your shift as much as possible.
- Have examples of practice documents or reports that you can use as templates.
- Take your breaks and recharge—this might include finding a quiet area to have your break or taking a walk. Don't be afraid to explain why you need to do this and not sit in a noisy staff area.
- Try to find somewhere quieter to write up notes; this could be by your patient's bedspace, the car if working in community or an office—this might be included in your reasonable adjustments for practice.
- Discuss using a device such as a phone as a timer/reminder/spell-checker/pronunciation helper/note taker/calculator. Make it clear why you want to use your device and use it professionally.
- Have a notebook or paper with you to write things down (remember, confidential information should be shredded at the end of the shift).
- Use an A-Z notebook to put in common drugs, normal observation ranges for common diseases or ages or anything else that you might want to know regularly but struggle to remember.
- Borrow equipment or book additional time in the skills lab so that you can practice clinical skills. Ask for extra help if you need it; it will also show your commitment to the course.

SOCIAL MEDIA
@susie_wilkie

'Just be you, keep your standards high and shout when you need help. Never feel less than, we all need time to settle into new roles and some things take longer than others'

What tools or tips will you try? What works for you and what did not work?

_____

_____

_____

_____

CASE STUDY

When I started the registered nurse degree apprenticeship, I spoke with my tutor about my suspicions of dyslexia, my previous experiences within primary school and the difficulties I face with academic work. I was provided a preassessment to complete, which determines the possibility of dyslexia. I scored a high probability, which led me to seek an accredited dyslexia assessor, supported by the university. I needed to travel off the island for the official assessment; however, this was supported by the university and concluded my dyslexia.

Since I have received my diagnosis, I have not needed to advocate for myself as much within the academic setting. The tutors at the university have been quicker to come forward and discuss the support needs I have, as the diagnosis is now officially attached to my student record. If I should need it, extra time for assignments can be provided, and currently, all module content is printed on paper. I found a mustard yellow promotes my concentration whilst reading material; it has been my favourite tool.

I have found within practice, there is more understanding from peers. I have seen a big difference with acceptance. People want to

CASE STUDY—cont'd

help more. It takes extra time for me to use textbooks or printed templates. A part of my reasonable adjustments to promote time management is the use of my mobile phone. I use the British National Formulary phone app to search medications, the NHS BMI checker as well as a spell checker to ensure correct documentation. Placement areas have also provided documentation for my review.

I find being open about my diagnosis can be challenging. You never know what response you are going to get. I received negative attitudes prediagnosis, which affected my confidence, and some people appear to be impartial with my diagnosis now. I have to remind myself, 'You cannot let one negative experience stop you from experiencing new opportunities'. Since my diagnosis, the positive experiences outweigh the negative. Not only has my diagnosis enabled me to understand more about myself, as well as dyslexia, I have received more understanding from others than not. I have access to more resources than I did prediagnosis, such as the reasonable adjustments. To help remove the stigma around neurodivergent conditions, I cofounded SSHINE (Sharing Student Healthcare Initiative for Neurodiversity and Equity). SSHINE is made up of MDT healthcare students.

Jade Wareham, registered nurse degree apprenticeship student

Maintaining your well-being

As highlighted in Chapter 1, your well-being and mental health as a nursing student are always important and arguable even more so if you are neurodivergent, as anxiety and depression have been found to co-occur more often. Nursing is a difficult programme, physically, psychologically and emotionally, and you need to look after yourself to be able to give the best to your patients. You may also have to work harder than others to keep up with the work or just to get through the day, and this can be exhausting and can lead to burnout or meltdowns.

Stress can also affect your performance more, and you might find that you are affected more by neurodivergent traits when you are stressed or tired; for example, if you have dyspraxia, you might find that you are clumsier or walk into things more or your working memory is worse (Major and Tetley, 2019).

TIP

Here are a few things that might help you:

- Seek help early. Avoiding the issue will not make it go away; it will only get worse. Identify what is making you feel stressed, anxious or sad, and try to take measures to address them. This might mean seeking support from the university mental health support team, disability team, your tutor or doctor.
- Avoid procrastination. You may well be very skilled at this, especially for tasks that you find difficult or boring, but this can lead to increased stress as deadlines approach. See Chapter 2 for further guidance on this.
- Try to get enough sleep, although this may not always be easy, as sleep problems can also be associated with neurodivergence. If this is the case, seek advice on sleep problems and try to maintain sleep hygiene and as much of a sleep routine as possible.
- Maintain a healthy lifestyle, eat well and exercise. Exercise can be particularly helpful for those with ADHD and can help focus as well as reducing stress.
- Consider mindfulness and meditation. For those who find this difficult, try practicing mindfulness during a walk or while moving.
- Maintain a work/life balance. You still need to have downtime and be able to relax.
- Take regular breaks when studying or in practice.
- Seek out a mentor or coach.
- Talk to friends or colleagues.

Connecting with others

Reaching out to others who are also neurodivergent can help you to learn and to share your experiences. You might have a neurodiversity network at university or just talk to someone else you know. Social media groups can be a useful source of peer support, and many have Twitter chats specifically around neurodiversity or offer tips, advice or mutual support.

SOCIAL MEDIA
@StNHeather

'Network with other neurodivergent students/staff. Find your own tribe that you can get support, give support and vent to/from to know you're not alone and increase each other's confidence. Finding people with lived experience is important'

Useful Twitter groups:

- @NDNursesUK
- @SSHINE_students
- @SUNN_project

What actions do you plan to take to maintain your well-being?

_____

_____

_____

_____

CONCLUSION

Remember that you have got to university on your own merits; you have worked hard and achieved a lot to get here and, in the process, developed a lot of skills and strategies that will help you to continue to progress. Use those strategies and develop new ones that will enable you to thrive at university and in practice. Look out for signs that you are struggling, and don't be afraid to ask for help or support and look after yourself. You have demonstrated resilience and determination, and that will take you far in your nursing career.

Now you have finished this chapter. Please make notes on what you have learned.

_____

_____

_____

_____

_____

_____

_____

_____

_____

_____

_____

_____

_____

_____

_____

_____

_____

_____

_____

REFERENCES

British Dyslexia Association (2010) Definition of dyslexia. Available at: https://www.bdadyslexia.org.uk/dyslexia/about-dyslexia/what-is-dyslexia

Disability Discrimination Act (1995) c.50 [online] Available at: https://www.legislation.gov.uk/ukpga/1995/50/

Equality Act (2010). C.15 [online] Available at: http://www.legislation.gov.uk/ukpga/2010/15

Focusmate (2023) The science behind Focusmate. Available at: https://www.focusmate.com/science

Lino, F., Chieffo, D.P.R. (2022) Developmental coordination disorder and most prevalent comorbidities: a narrative review. Children, 9, 1095. Available at: https:// doi.org/10.3390/children9071095

Major, R., Tetley, J. (2019) Effects of dyslexia on registered nurses in practice. Nurse Education in Practice Vol. 35 p7-13

Matthews, B., Redstone, R. and Lord, Z. (2019) Dyslexia – be proud of your difference, by Ruth May, Chief Nursing Officer for England, Available at: https://blog.horizonsnhs.com/post/102fs4n/dyslexia-be-proud-of-your-difference-by-ruth-may-chief-nursing-officer-for-eng

Microsoft (2023) Accessibility tools for neurodiversity. Available at: https://support.microsoft.com/en-gb/topic/accessibility-tools-for-neurodiversity-6dbd8065-b543-4cf8-bdfb-7c84d9e8f74a

National Institute for Health and Care Excellence (NICE) (2022) Attention deficit hyperactivity disorder: How common is it? Available at: https://cks.nice.org.uk/topics/attention-deficit-hyperactivity-disorder/background-information/prevalence/

Neurodiversity Celebration Week (2023) What is neurodiversity? Available at: https:// www.neurodiversityweek.com/introduction

Nursing and Midwifery Council (2018a) Standards of proficiency for registered nurses. Available at: https://www.nmc.org.uk/standards/standards-for-nurses/

Nursing and Midwifery Council (2018b) The code: professional standards of practice and behaviour for nurses, midwives and nursing associates. Available at: https:// www.nmc.org.uk/standards/code/

Rose, J. (2009) Identifying and teaching children and young people with dyslexia and literacy difficulties, Available at: http://www.thedyslexia-spldtrust.org.uk/media/downloads/inline/the-rose-report.1294933674.pdf

Royal College of Nursing (no date) Neurodiversity guidance. Available at: https://www.rcn.org.uk/get-help/member-support-services/peer-support-services/neurodiversity-guidance